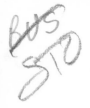
What's
New
in
Allergy

Other Books by the Author

Hidden Food Allergies; How to Find and Overcome Them Successfully

Take Charge of Your Health: Professional Secrets You Need to Know to Obtain the Best Medical Care

THIRD EDITION, UPDATED AND REVISED

What's New in Allergy

NEW DEVELOPMENTS
AND HOW THEY
HELP YOU OVERCOME
ALLERGY AND ASTHMA

Stephen Astor, M.D.

Printed in the United States of America.

10 9 8 7 6 5 4 3 2

Cataloging Data

Astor, Stephen, date.
What's New In Allergy.
216p.   22.6cm.
Index.
1. Health   2. Self-care, Health   3. Medicine, Popular
4. Consumer education   5. Medical care   6. Alternative medicine.
number   1992   616.97   91-91432
ISBN 091500108X

Table of Contents

Introduction 1

1 How People Get Allergies 5
Now We Understand Why People Suddenly Develop
   Allergies 6
How Allergies Run In Families 8
Can Breast Feeding Prevent Allergy? 9

2 Newly Discovered Allergens and Chemical Mediators 11
Discovery That Vitamins Can Cause Allergic Reactions 12
Natural Healthy Carrots Cause Allergy 13
A Bodily Chemical Is Found To Be Responsible For
   Allergic Reactions 14

3 Food Additives 19
Treatment For Food Additive Allergy 20
Dr. Feingold Denies That Food Additives Cause
   Hyperactivity 21

4 Food Allergy 25
Sugar Allergy Findings 26
Good News For Kids With Food Allergies 27
New Drug For Food Allergy 28
Milk Allergy Shown To Cause Arthritis 30
Migraine Headaches Due To Food Allergy And Pseudo Food
   Allergy 31
A Word About Avoidance Of Foods 32

5 Allergy To Pets 33
Cat Hair Doesn't Cause Allergy 34
No One Is Safe From Dogs And Cats 34
Washing Cats Removes Allergenic Dander 35
Allergy Injections For Cats And Dogs 36

6 Mold Allergy........ 39
Mold Is In The Kitchen 40
Heat Kills Mold 40

7 Allergy Testing 43
How To Reduce The Number Of Allergy Tests For Airborne
Allergens........ 44
Inaccuracy Of Food Tests Confirmed........ 45
Three Blood Tests For Allergy........ 47

8 Allergy Injections 55
The One-Shot Cure For Allergies........ 56
New Type Of Allergy Injections Means Fewer Shots
(Polymerized Extract) 60
Polymerized Serum May Not Be Better Than Traditional
Serum 64
Pollen Can Bother You After The Pollen Season Ends........ 65
Shots For Severe Asthma Attacks........ 65
Discovery That Allergy Serum Loses Potency Quickly........ 66
Dust Mite In Your Allergy Serum Can Ruin Your Chance
For Successful Immunization........ 68
New Explanation For Injection Failure With Ragweed
Allergy 69
Oral Drops Might Replace Allergy Injections........ 70
How Often To Repeat Skin Tests 71

9 Medications Which Alleviate Allergy........ 75
Antihistamines Can Make Asthma Worse........ 76
New Antihistamine Doesn't Make You Sleepy........ 77
The Newest New Antihistamine That Doesn't Make
You Sleepy 80
Twenty-Four Hour Antihistamine 82
Six Kinds Of Adverse Reactions To Drugs........ 83
How Vitamin C Was Thought To Help Allergies........ 84
Theophylline Can Cause Emotional Problems In
Children 86
Tests For Theophylline Drug Level........ 87

Breaking Asthma Tablets To Obtain Half-Doses Can Be
   Dangerous... 88
Albuterol Powder And Ketotifen--Two New Drugs For
   Asthma 89
Vomiting And Nausea From Allergy Medicines 90
Beta Blockers Can Make Asthma Worse............................ 92

10 Nasal Sprays... 93
Nasal Sprays For Allergy 93
Unpleasant Side Effect Of Nasal Inhalers 99

11 Asthma.. 101
Anti-inflammatory Drugs Are The Hot Treatment For
   Asthma 102
Delayed Asthma Reactions 103
Risk of Developing Asthma In Occupations Where
   There Is Exposure To Animals..................................... 104
Sinus Infections Can Cause Asthma..................................105
Asthma-Provoking Chemical Found In Medicine
   Used To Treat Asthma 106
Sudden Fatal Asthma With Open Airways 107
Inhalation Technique For Asthmatics................................108
Spacers For Steroid/Cortisone Inhalers............................ 110
Overdiagnosis And Overtreatment Of Black Asthmatics..110
Negative Ion Generators For Treating Asthma..................111
Discovery Of What Provokes Asthma After Exercise........ 112
Exercise-Induced Asthma Is Unrecognized.......................114
Asthma Worse If Family Member Smokes.........................115
Long-Lasting Inhaler For Asthma 116
Peak-Flow Meters..117

12 Allergy And Pregnancy 119
Asthma Symptoms During Pregnancy...............................119
Allergy Injections Do Not Sensitize The Fetus..................120
Fetus Protected Against Allergy When Mother
   Gets Shots..121

13 Penicillin Allergy............ 123
Penicilin Allergy No Longer a Widespread Threat............ 124
Tests For Penicillin Allergy............ 125
Testing For Penicillin Allergy Has Limited Value............ 126

14 Bee Sting Allergy............ 129
Bee Sting Injections Need Not Last Forever............ 130
Killer Bee Threat Is Overdramatized............ 131

15 New Diseases............ 133
Hives And Swelling During Exercise............ 133
Exercise Can Be Harmful............ 134
Trigger Of Chronic Hives............ 135
Definition Of Chronic Hives............ 135
Occupational Allergies............ 136

16 House Dust Control and The Home Environment............ 141
House Dust Mite Allergy............ 141
Effectiveness Of Air Cleaners............ 143
Facts on Exposure To Home Insulation............ 144

17 Miscellaneous............ 147
Hope For Sinus Headache Sufferers............ 148
Treatment Found For Itchy, Watery Eyes............ 149
How To Avoid Allergens............ 149
Why Allergy Symptoms Are Often Worse At Night............ 152
Surprising Death From Bee Pollen............ 153
Discovery Of The Worst Location In The United States
    For Allergy Sufferers............ 154
Discovery Of The Worst Year For Allergy Sufferers............ 156
Treatment For Allergy To X-Ray Contrast Material............ 158
Latex Glove Skin Reactions............ 158
Wife Allergic To Husband............ 159

18 Not New, But Worth Remembering............161
The One-Visit Allergy Workup.............162
The Three Treatments For Allergy.............162
The Best Way To Take Cortisone (Steroids).............165
Will The Real Allergist Please Stand Up?.............170

19 Problems And Deception In Allergy.............177
Questions To Ask About A New Treatment Or Theory....178
Serious Deficiencies That Have Been Noted In The
   Treatment Of Asthma.............179
Total Environmental Allergy And Clinical Ecology.............182
Monday Morning Sickness.............183

20 The Future of Allergy.............185
Histamine Releasing Factor Has Been Found To Be
   Responsible For Allergies.............186
Exciting And Revolutionary Treatment For Allergies.......186
Another New Treatment For Allergy.............187
A Science Fiction Proposal For An Allergy Cure.............188

Appendix A.............191
Partial List of Drugs Used in Allergy Treatment

Appendix B.............197
Other Books About Allergy

Index.............199

Introduction

Mitch was an eager college student who wanted to make his fortune early in life. As soon as he graduated from the university, he entered a training program to learn how to sell stocks and bonds. At his one-month review the training director praised Mitch's progress, but he also issued a warning. "Mitch," he said, "you can't deal with the public effectively if you're constantly blowing your nose and clearing your throat."

"I can't help it." Mitch replied. "I have terrible allergy."

"Why don't you get some treatment?" the director asked. "You'd make a much better impression."

"What's the use?" Mitch answered. "Allergy treatment hasn't changed in ages. They can't cure you."

Mitch expressed a typical viewpoint. Many people believe there is nothing new in allergy. The facts are quite the opposite.

During the last few years, there has been an explosion of information about how allergy affects your body. This has led to better control of allergy through more advanced medication, refinement in the way injections are given, better understanding of food allergy, and simplified ways to avoid allergenic substances.

This book, *What's New in Allergy*, describes the pros and cons of the new developments.

You hear and read a lot about allergy on radio, in magazines, and in newspaper articles, but you don't usually find a balanced discussion. Radio, newspapers and magazines need to grab your attention. So, what they tell you is ordinarily lopsided one way or the other. They report the views of those who are eager to promote a certain treatment and thus emphasize the advantages. Or, they feature stories which quote those who oppose a treatment and emphasize the disadvantages. As is often the case, the truth is somewhere in between.

By understanding both sides of the different claims about allergy treatment, you can determine for yourself whether a new finding, drug, machine, or injection is suitable for *you*.

> *What is true for one person is not necessarily true for another.*

In this book, each significant development is explained in easy to understand language. You may read the entire book or simply turn to the section that fits your case.

I divided the book into chapters. Each chapter contains several reports. Each report describes the results of experiments that have been performed by experts in the field of allergy. To give you an example, at the last annual meeting of the American Academy of Allergy and Immunology scientists discussed over eight hundred experiments. This gives you an idea of the enormous amount of research taking place in the field of allergy. And, the American Academy of Allergy and Immunology is just one of many allergy associations.

Although I don't discuss complex, biochemical reactions in this book, the study of basic mechanisms is vitally important. Doctors hope fundamental research will one day lead to a permanent cure.

The studies I describe are more practical. They deal with how and when to use new drugs, ways to improve the effectiveness of injections, measures that have been found helpful in preventing allergies, and certain diseases whose origin was unknown but, upon investigation, turned out to be caused by allergy. Equally important for you, and often overlooked, are studies which show the limitations and disadvantages of allergy treatments that were once thought to be useful and have now been shown to be ineffective or dangerous.

From their research, doctors understand such facts as why people inherit allergies and what causes allergy symptoms. You will be surprised to learn that allergy is not a deficiency or defect in the body but an overabundance of a particular antibody, called IgE.

The section on drugs explains how to utilize the new drugs to achieve their optimum effect. You will also learn simple techniques to avoid allergens so that you can prevent your allergy symptoms from even starting.

There is a lot of information packed into these pages. Some of it is so new your doctors may not even know about it. Physicians who are in clinical practice often don't have the time to read about advances in *every* field of medicine. That is why there are specialists. Specialists concentrate on one field. If your doctor wants to know more about a particular topic, I included the name of at least one of the scientists who did the original research. Thus, your doctor can read the original experiment.

At the end of each report you will find helpful hints to aid you in putting the information into perspective. An allergy treatment that applies to women may not apply to men. A treatment that works in children may not help adults. An injection for pollens may not help food allergy. A technique that seems to cure allergy quickly may have long-term side effects.

Unfortunately, there isn't a universal answer that fits every situation. This is why you need to understand as much as you can. This is the only way you will obtain the best treatment *for your particular problem.*

Know What You Are Doing To Your Body

When you suffer from a chronic disease such as allergy, you should learn the advantages and disadvantages of any treatment prescribed for you. You may not like what you hear, however. Sometimes the truth is hard to take. But it's better for you to face the facts from the beginning. Where your health is concerned, improper treatment can be more than a mere disappointment. It can actually harm you!

What's New in Allergy is an adventure. Your trip will unmask myths, teach you surprising facts, and help *you,* the allergy sufferer, get the most from modern medicine.

1

How People
Get Allergies

There are a lot of myths and misunderstandings about how people develop allergy. Over the years I've encountered them all. For example, you may have heard allergy is a weakness or deficiency of your immune system. Or, you may have have been told allergy is from lack of vitamins or too much histamine.

Although people have different ideas about what causes allergy, their reaction upon being told allergy is responsible for their symptoms is usually the same. "I don't believe it. How could I suddenly be allergic to a substance I've been eating or exposed to my whole life?"

The first two studies explain how allergies begin and how they run in families. After doctors understood how allergies developed, they turned their attention to devising a way to prevent allergies. So, the last study describes the results of an experiment that was done in the expectation that you could prevent allergy from developing by breast-feeding your children.

Now We Understand Why People Suddenly Develop Allergies

You may be puzzled about how you could suddenly be allergic to a dog you've had for ten years or a cheese you've been eating for twenty years. The symptoms seem to appear out of the clear blue sky. And, because there were no prior indications of allergy, you may not believe this could be happening to you.

Although a sudden onset of symptoms may seem unique to allergy, the process occurs with many diseases. Cancer, heart conditions, and ulcer are typical examples. These illnesses develop over a period of time. But you only become aware you've developed one of these illnesses at a specific point in time.

This is the story with allergic disorders. Certain people are *predisposed* to allergy due to a flaw in their ability to regulate the level of an antibody called IgE. Because of this flaw, they eventually make *too much* IgE. Slowly and surely and after repeated exposure to various substances, their level of IgE rises. When their IgE has reached a level that is excessive, the actual symptoms begin. Dr. Rebecca Buckley of Duke University studied IgE and confirmed that allergy is due to excess IgE antibody.

> *Once IgE hits an excess level, the symptoms of allergy begin.*

Those of you who manufacture IgE very fast will reach an excess level early in your life and therefore develop allergies when you are young. Those of you who manufacture IgE more slowly might take fifteen or twenty years to reach an excess level. Some of you, and this is true of the majority of individuals, manufacture IgE at the normal rate and, lucky you, you *never* develop allergies.

Exposure Needed For Allergy To Develop

There is an additional fact you need to know to help you understand why allergies take time to develop. Your body won't make antibodies unless it is exposed to a particular substance. For example, if you never take penicillin, you could not become allergic to penicillin. However, if your body has the tendency or predisposition to make too much IgE antibody and if you take a lot of penicillin, chances are you'll eventually wind up allergic to penicillin. The same is true for exposure to grasses, weeds, trees, dust, and dogs.

In fact, when it comes to determining what is most likely responsible for the apparent sudden onset of allergic symptoms, most allergists are more suspicious of substances you've been exposed to throughout your life than something that is brand new in your life.

Helpful hint 1: Allergies develop over a period of time after repeated exposure in certain susceptible individuals.

Helpful hint 2: Two thirds of people manufacture IgE antibody at the *normal* rate. No matter how often these individuals are exposed to allergenic substances they *never* become allergic. Population studies show that the *remaining* one-third of the population has allergy. In these studies, though, allergy is defined in strict medical terms (i.e. excess IgE). People who are allergic to work or their spouse don't count!

Helpful hint 3: Even though one third of people develop allergy, many cases are mild and do not need extensive treatment.

How Allergies Run In Families

As you may have heard, allergies tend to occur in families. This is because the difficulty in regulating IgE antibody is usually an *inherited* characteristic.

Interestingly, individual members of a family don't inherit allergy to the *same* substance. Since they inherit the *predisposition to develop* allergy, what they actually become allergic to depends on their lifestyles and habits, since these determine the degree of their exposure to various allergens.

Dr. Sami Bahna thought it would be a good idea to study twins to learn which specific allergies occur in families.

Studies Of Twins

Dr. Bahna showed that if one twin had allergies, the other did too. However, the specific allergens each twin was allergic to and the way those allergens affected them were different.

If one twin was allergic to grasses and weeds, the other could be allergic to dogs and cats. One to foods and the other to dust. To make it more confusing, if both twins were allergic to dog dander, in one the dog could provoke sneezing and in the other it could provoke wheezing. In one of them peanuts could cause hives, while in the other peanuts might provoke gastrointestinal symptoms. There was no way Dr. Bahna could predict how one twin would react no matter how extensively he studied the other.

Dr. Bahna's research is a good reminder that when individuals inherit allergy, they inherit the *ability to become allergic* and not allergy to a specific substance.

Helpful hint 1: The *predisposition* to develop allergy runs in families. Allergy to a *specific substance* is determined by exposure to those substances.

Helpful hint 2: You cannot skin test one member of your family in order to learn about the allergies of the other members of your family.

Can Breast Feeding Prevent Allergies?

Since doctors know that allergy is caused by exposure to substances *and* the inherited tendency to make excessive IgE, they theorized that by removing the exposure side of the equation they might be able to prevent the accumulation of excess IgE.

To investigate this, Dr. Robert Hamburger from San Diego studied breast-feeding, which is a natural, everyday experiment. Dr. Hamburger divided women into two groups. Some breast-fed their babies, and some did not. If the breast-fed children had grown up free of allergy, the answer would have been clear-cut. However, when the results were in, some of the children who were breast-fed got allergy anyway. Of the bottle-fed children, some didn't get allergy.

When you think about how complicated the allergic process is, you'd expect this sort of result. Since it takes exposure *and* susceptibility to produce allergy, removing only one of the factors, the exposure to cows' milk, would simply *delay* an infant's exposure and subsequent sensitization. Breast-feeding could not be expected to prevent allergy to milk *forever*. Even if avoiding cows' milk was successful in preventing allergy to cow's milk, this would not prevent a child's exposure to other foods. Nor would it prevent exposure to dust, grasses, or a family dog.

Aside from the theoretical arguments against this idea, the most telling blow and the most important consideration was that the experiment just did not work.

The basic defect in allergy is an inherited characteristic, much like the color of your eyes is an inherited characteristic. And, you cannot change your inheritance by changing your diet.

Additionally, a more recent study by Dr. S. Giordano showed that when a nursing mother eats foods, the foods can pass into the breast milk where they are ingested by and therefore sensitize susceptible infants. So, breast-feeding alone is not guaranteed to prevent allergies.

Helpful hint 1: Breast-feeding can *delay* the exposure of your infant to cows' milk. However, if you eat cows' milk while breast-feeding, you may pass enough cows' milk protein to your infant through your breast milk so that your infant becomes allergic anyway.

Helpful hint 2: Breast-feeding does not prevent or delay exposure to other allergens such as dogs, cats, dust, pollens, and other foods. Even if it could, you cannot keep your babies in protective custody for their whole life.

Helpful hint 3: Whether you breast-feed or not, only one third of children develop allergy anyway.

Helpful hint 4: If your child develops allergy, you can begin treatment at any time. Usually, treatment requires only a few simple changes in the environment.

Helpful hint 5: If you want to breast feed because you enjoy it, go right ahead. If you're breast-feeding to prevent allergies, you should reconsider your decision.

2

Newly Discovered Allergens and Chemical Mediators

Doctors already have enough trouble treating allergens such as dogs, cats, grasses, trees, and weeds, so you may wonder why they make more work for themselves by looking for *additional* allergens to treat. Unless your doctors are aware of *all* the possibilities, they might overlook an allergen that may be crucial in *your* particular case. Two of the following studies tell you about substances that were previously unsuspected as causes of allergy. One substance is a vitamin. The other is a healthy, natural food.

Allergens are substances *outside* your body which initiate allergic reactions. However, they need the cooperation of substances, called chemical mediators, which are substances made *within* your body. These *internal* chemicals trigger the actual symptoms you feel.

Thus, doctors need to learn as much about chemical mediators as about allergens. This improves their ability to alleviate your symptoms. For example, almost everyone has heard that histamine, which is made in Mast cells in your tissues, is responsible for causing allergy symptoms. But other bodily chemicals are just as deleterious. So, the last study tells you about new chemical mediators that have been found to be the root cause of allergy.

Discovery That Vitamins Can Cause Allergic Reactions

Vitamins are supposed to be beneficial and harmless to the human body. So, the discovery that a vitamin could give you allergy was a shock. Dr. Jerry Dolovich from Canada treated a man who collapsed and had seizures after taking a vitamin tablet. The man had such a severe reaction he wound up in an intensive care unit.

After a great deal of investigation, Dr. Dolovich and his co-workers uncovered the culprit. This was polyethylene glycol, a chemical that is found in many medicinal tablets. Polyethylene glycol is used to bind different ingredients in many common tablets.

This shows that you never know how or where allergy will strike. Even something as harmless as a vitamin tablet may contain an ingredient that can cause a severe reaction.

Helpful hint 1: Allergy reactions can occur in the most unexpected circumstances, so you have to be careful.

Helpful hint 2: Many people claim they are allergic to various drugs when in fact they aren't allergic to the active ingredient in the tablet but to one of the other substances in the tablet.

Helpful hint 3: Just for fun, I thought you might be interested in seeing a list of various ingredients commonly used to manufacture tablets. It's astounding to learn that when you purchase a drug for its active ingredient, you are getting a whole bunch of other substances too.

• Fillers-- an ingredient that fills tablets or capsules (e.g., dicalcium phosphate, vegetable oil).
• Binders-- a substance that holds tablets together (e.g., lactose, cornstarch).
• Lubricant-- a chemical that allows tablets to be ejected from the compression mold (e.g., magnesium stearate).
• Glidant-- an ingredient that prevents blended material from clumping (e.g., a mineral from hydrated silica).
• Disintegrant-- a substance that makes tablets break apart in the digestive tract (e.g., starch).
• Coating-- a chemical that protects tablets from light or moisture (e.g., sugar).
• Flavors and Sweeteners-- substances that are found in chewable and liquid drugs (e.g., fructose, sorbitol).
• Colors-- a chemical used for identification. This can be natural or artificial (e.g., carotene, tartrazine).

Natural Healthy Carrots Cause Allergy

Dr. S. Lehrer from New Orleans treated a patient who developed swelling of the throat and difficulty breathing within minutes after eating a carrot. Since carrots are supposed to be healthy and full of vitamins, this was hard to believe. But on subsequent testing the person reacted each time, thus proving that carrots can be healthy for some and nearly deadly for others.

Helpful hint 1: Even natural, healthy foods can be bad for you if you're allergic to them.

A Bodily Chemical Is Found To Be Responsible For Allergic Reactions
(Or, The Real Story Why Antihistamines Don't Always Work.)

After hearing so much about IgE causing allergy, you may feel cheated to learn that I only told you half the story. Your body also needs *chemical mediators*. Unlike IgE, which must be present in excess, you need only average, everyday amounts of chemical mediators to cause your allergy symptoms.

Chemical mediators are made and stored in various cells. Ordinarily they are released in small amounts as they're required for normal, physiologic function. However, if you have too much IgE antibody, your body loses control of the way those chemicals are released.

The most well known of the chemical mediators is histamine. Patients often ask if they are allergic because they have too much histamine in their bodies. Strictly speaking, an allergic individual is *not* overflowing with histamine. Your cells contain just the normal amount. But, if your cells release histamine at inappropriate times, your symptoms occur.

> *It's not too much histamine but rather the inappropriate release of histamine that causes allergy symptoms.*

Other Bodily Chemicals That Contribute To Allergy

Below is a list of other chemicals that are important to your body but can contribute to allergy symptoms. Like histamine, these, too, can be inappropriately released under the proper conditions. When this occurs, they can provoke your symptoms. Dr. Frank Austen, who has done a lot of research in this area, is an articulate lecturer on this subject.

Histamine
SRS-A
HETE
PGD
Prostaglandin
Leukotriene
TAME esterase activity
Kinin
Bradykinin
Lysyl Bradykinin
PAF (platelet activating factor)
Thromboxane
Major Basic Protein
Histamine Releasing Factors
Interferon
Interleukin

Although these names are long, difficult to pronounce, and probably boring to you, allergists are excited when they read about them. Once doctors learn which chemical mediator is responsible for a particular symptom, the drug companies can discover an antidote, just like *anti*histamine is the antidote for histamine.

Many times I have wished histamine was the only chemical mediator we had to deal with, because we already have the antidote for it. Unfortunately, the other chemicals on the list are responsible for just as many allergic reactions as histamine. This explains why antihistamines alone don't always help you.

Misleading Reports About Allergy Cures

When it comes to believing the medical reports that you read in newspapers and magazines, you must be cautious. Certain newspaper reporters don't have the technical expertise to evaluate medical information, so they frequently rely on a person who is enthusiastic but biased about a particular research study's findings. In the field of allergy, chemical mediators are sometimes subject to this kind of twisted reporting.

Over the years I've read many feature stories that would make you think a miracle cure for allergy was around the corner. In their zeal to create eye-catching headlines, some reporters ignore the words of cautious doctors who try to explain when a discovery is just a preliminary finding.

Allergy researchers are constantly finding chemical mediators. So far, though, no chemical mediator is *solely* responsible for every type of allergic condition. The dominant chemical mediator that causes sneezing in one individual is usually different from the one that causes sneezing in another individual. To make matters more complicated, it is usually a *combination* of chemical mediators that causes sneezing in a particular individual. This kind of subtle information is not good for headlines.

Even when doctors isolate chemical mediators and demonstrate that they are responsible for allergic reactions, the doctors still have to invent drugs to counteract the mediators. Even if they could do that, they would then need to test the drugs for safety in children, adults, and pregnant women. Then they'd have to figure out which drug works for a particular individual without producing serious side effects.

At this stage of my medical career, it's too much for me to believe doctors will soon have a single, magic pill that works for all of you.

Additionally, none of the mediators on the above list are *truly* new, unless in your mind "new" covers the last five to ten years. The mediators that have captured the media's fancy are interleukins, leukotrienes, TAME esterase activity, and Histamine Releasing Factors. After years studying these so-called new mediators, though, the final verdict is still not in. So, I'm sorry to say this, but when you read of the next latest breakthrough in finding "the cause" of allergy, don't get your hopes too high.

Helpful hint 1: Several normal chemicals made by the human body participate in causing allergic reactions. Although these chemicals are important for your everyday physiologic function, the cells of allergic patients release these chemicals inappropriately. This results in allergy symptoms.

Helpful hint 2: There have been no truly new chemicals discovered in many years. But doctors are learning new things about the ones that have already been found.

Helpful hint 3: Hopefully, understanding the many interactions between chemical mediators, IgE, and allergens such as dogs, dust, and pollens, will enable your doctors to control your allergies better.

3

Food Additive Allergy

Foods are a well-known cause of allergy symptoms. This is not new information to you. Even in ancient times people experienced reactions to foods.

The twentieth century simply added a new dimension to the problem. In order to transport foods, keep them fresh, and make them appeal to your sense of taste, sight, and smell, manufacturers had to add chemicals during the processing procedure. Thus, they created a modern allergy problem.

You may have heard stories of reactions to food additives. However, you can't believe everything you hear. The following two studies illustrate true and false reports.

In one case, food additives were proven to provoke problems. In the other case, although the problem exists, it seems to have been blown out of proportion. See Appendix B for a suggestion about additional reading on the subject of food allergy.

Treatment For Food Additive Allergy

There is a form of asthma where, upon eating a salad in a restaurant, you may experience an attack of asthma. The salad literally takes your breath away. Some individuals with this susceptibility also break out in hives from head to foot. These reactions are dramatic, severe, and can be difficult to stop. In a few cases they've led to a fatality.

This type of sensitivity is due to a preservative called bisulfite and is said to occur in one out of ten asthmatic adults. Although allergists have known about this kind of reaction for years, they haven't found a simple solution other than to recommend avoidance.

In certain people there are similar reactions to aspirin, a yellow food dye called tartrazine, pain killers, and several anti-inflammatory drugs such as Naprosyn, Motrin, and Ibuprofen.

It is upsetting to me that newspaper and TV reporters often blow the problem out of proportion. They make you think everyone in the United States reacts to these chemicals. In fact, only a few individuals are affected. For those of you who are susceptible, of course, this is a serious problem. For the rest of you, though, this is not a concern. And, there is no evidence that ingestion of these types of chemicals makes you become allergic to them, unless you are a predisposed individual.

Those who have such reactions should avoid the chemicals. This is the safest policy. But, Dr. Donald Stevenson at Scripps Clinic in La Jolla, California, is working on a way to treat such individuals for the aspirin-salicylate kind of chemical sensitivity by administering medication to desensitize them. He's studying the exact dose and timing that's needed to accomplish this. And, allergists in clinical practice hope he'll finish soon. Allergists in practice also hope he'll find something for the bisulfite and yellow dye sufferers too.

Additional Help Is On The Way

In 1986 the United States Food and Drug Administration acknowledged the problem of sulfite sensitivity and banned the use of these types of chemicals on fresh fruit and vegetables. The FDA also required that packages be labelled when they contain certain levels of sulfites. But you should not depend on voluntary compliance with these rules by restaurants and supermarkets. The consequences of a mistake can endanger your life.

Helpful hint 1: If you have aspirin sensitivity, there is a possibility you can be desensitized.

Helpful hint 2: When you read or hear any medical warning, ask what percent of people have the problem. You must keep fearful news in perspective and not become paranoid over each ominous report that appears in newspapers, magazines, and television.

Helpful hint 3: If you are sensitive to sulfites, you cannot trust that every restaurant in the United States knows about and complies with the 1986 FDA ban on sulfites.

Dr. Ben Feingold Denies That Food Additives Cause Hyperactivity

For many years I had heard that Dr. Ben Feingold believed food additives and preservatives could cause hyperactivity, especially in children. Dr. Feingold was a pioneer in allergy and contributed a great deal to our understanding of the allergic process. But, his diet theory was controversial since other scientists could not prove his ideas were unequivocally true.

Scientists are trained to think in terms of constant laws. When Isaac Newton stated he had discovered a law of gravity which proved that objects are pulled toward the center of the earth, other scientists would have found it hard to accept Newton's law if it did not work twenty-four hours a day. They would have ridiculed gravity that one day pulled objects toward earth and another day sent the same objects shooting into space.

Dr. Feingold's diet theory ran afoul of scientists' expectations for consistency and constancy. Not every patient with hyperactivity improved when they followed the Feingold diet. In fact, only a few people benefited.

On the other hand, if the Feingold diet helped only one out of ten people this meant the diet was partially successful. So, you need to work with your doctors to determine whether you are a responder or a non-responder. There are many medical treatments where results cannot be guaranteed since no two individuals are alike in every respect.

In addition to the diet's being unable to guarantee relief in every case, just the symptoms the diet was meant to alleviate were sometimes confusing. As I mentioned above, I had been under the impression from talking to many physicians and patients that the Feingold diet was supposed to help *hyper*activity. One day I came across a statement that claimed Dr. Feingold had said his diet did *not* reduce hyperactivity in children. I couldn't believe this so I wrote Dr. Feingold to ask if he had been quoted correctly. To my surprise he told me he had.

In his letter Dr. Feingold stated that his experience showed coloring agents, when added to foods, can cause *hypo*activity in children. This, as you probably know, is the exact opposite of *hyper*activity.

Helpful hint 1: According to Dr. Ben Feingold, food additives can cause *hypo*-activity, in certain individuals.

Helpful hint 2: Even when you think you understand a person's ideas, you sometimes need to ask a second time to be certain you understand *exactly* what they mean.

4

Food Allergy

Food allergy can cause many different symptoms. However, sometimes physicians don't even consider reactions to foods as a possibility when trying to make a diagnosis. This is unfortunate. In medicine, health care professionals need to have an open mind. By prejudging the diagnosis without backup data, a doctor could reach the wrong conclusion and therefore prescribe ineffective treatment.

Of course patients can err, too. Some of you may be too hasty in concluding foods are responsible for a particular problem. On the other hand, some of you may be too stubborn to look into the possibility.

The first two studies show you cannot assume you are allergic to foods. You must do a careful test to be sure. The third study describes a drug that can alleviate certain types of food allergy. The fourth shows that food allergy can cause arthritis, which was a completely unexpected finding. The next study explains how food can cause migraine headaches. And finally, there is a word about avoidance of foods.

Sugar Allergy Findings

Dr. Kathy Mahan studied sixteen children who had been diagnosed by their doctors as allergic to sugar. She hoped to learn what kinds of symptoms occurred and how she could help such patients.

When Dr. Mahan fed the sixteen children sugar-containing foods such as candy, the behavior of nine of the sixteen did not change. They did not become aggressive, overly active, loud, or argumentative. The remaining seven had a 15 percent increase in their activity level, but this was not much of a difference.

Being a good scientist, Dr. Mahan wanted to prove the seven who reacted were not cheating so she put sugar in capsules, in order to disguise the sugar taste. Then she fed the capsules to the children she was studying. Much to her dismay, none of the children reacted. This showed that the children had reacted only when they knew they were expected to react.

Thus, her experiment was a failure. She could not find children who were truly allergic to sugar.

In conclusion, Dr. Mahan observed that half of the children she had studied did not react *even when they knew* they were eating sugar. The other half reacted *only if they knew* they were eating sugar.

Helpful hint 1: It's easy for you or your doctors to blame bad behavior on sugar allergy. Whether you are corect or not is an entirely different matter.

Helpful hint 2: There may be rare individuals who react badly to sugar, but Dr. Kathy Mahan has shown that sugar allergy is very much over-diagnosed. Her experiment should make us pause to ask why people are so eager to blame difficult behavior problems in children, or even in themselves, on a food substance such as sugar instead of trying to figure out the real cause.

Good News For Kids With Food Allergies

For the past ten years Dr. Allan Bock has studied food allergy in children. His research is full of good news.

For three years he kept track of 500 children who were three years of age or under. He found that 40 percent of them (about 200 children) were reported by their parents and doctors to have had food reactions.

Of these 200 children, 33 percent (65 of the 200) proved allergic to fruits. These reactions were brief, usually lasting only a few hours. Twelve percent (26 children) reacted to milk, soybean, peanut, egg, wheat or chocolate. The remaining 55 perecent (109 children) did not react to anything. The diagram below illustrates this.

200 Children *Reported* Allergic

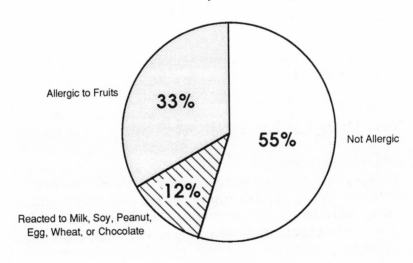

Just one year later when Dr. Bock reviewed those children who had reacted, he found they were no longer allergic. The offending food had been re-introduced into their diet without ill effect.

Helpful hint 1: Of all the children under three who are believed by their parents and doctors to have food allergies, 33 percent of these children are allergic just to fruits. However, their sensitivity doesn't usually last more than a few months. Twelve percent of these children are allergic to milk, soy, peanut, egg, wheat, or chocolate. And, 55 percent aren't allergic to anything. These 55 percent are being misdiagnosed.

Helpful hint 2: A lot of parents, doctors, or both are incorrectly blaming foods for causing symptoms in children.

Helpful hint 3: Even when foods cause allergy symptoms, the foods can almost always be re-introduced into the diet after a few months without causing adverse problems.

Helpful hint 4: Most children who are thought to have food allergy do not have food allergy.

New Drug For Food Allergy

When people react to a food, they commonly say they're allergic to the food. However, some of their reactions are due to poisoning such as from bacteria. Other reactions are due to an enzyme deficiency where the body can't digest a sugar, called lactose, which is found in milk products.

Others experience a metabolic type reaction such as the headaches that occur from Tyramine in cheese.

You may think I believe the number of people who have food allergy is minimal. The contrary is true. I believe *many* individuals suffer from food allergy. However, these individuals are often unaware that food can cause a multitude of symptoms and never investigate this possibility, thus overlooking an opportunity to determine the cause of their health problems.

Furthermore, there are many people who know they have food allergy, but don't know that something can be done about it.

Foods can cause a variety of conditions. You can determine whether you suffer from food allergy without going through expensive and inaccurate tests. In the field of food allergy there are many myths and misunderstandings that you should be aware of or else you'll wind up with inappropriate tests and useless treatment. To expose the myths and explain about food allergy, I wrote *Hidden Food Allergies*. See Appendix B for reading about food allergy.

If you've determined that you have food allergy after *proper* investigation, the best treatment is avoidance. In some cases there is another possibility. Some of you may be able to take a drug called cromolyn sodium prior to eating and *prevent* your food reactions.

The brand name of the drug is Gastrocrom. As usual, you won't know whether this medication works for you until you try it, but it is certainly worth trying. If you can prevent uncomfortable food reactions, you will be much happier.

Helpful hint 1: The key to treatment of food reactions is correct diagnosis of the type of reaction. Treatment of one type as if it were another is doomed to failure.

Helpful hint 2: If food allergy is responsible for certain symptoms, you *might* obtain relief by taking a new drug called Gastrocrom.

Helpful hint 3: Many food reactions are blamed on allergy when in fact the reactions are due to other mechanisms.

Milk Allergy Shown To Cause Arthritis

Dr. Richard Panush at the University of Florida discovered an amazing food reaction. He found an elderly woman who suffered from arthritis due to ingestion of milk.

Over the years there have been numerous claims in health books, magazines, newspaper articles, and even among certain health care professionals that food allergy can cause arthritis. However, the majority of experiments which supposedly proved that foods trigger arthritis were so poorly done that no scientist in good conscience could believe them.

Dr. Panush's study is believable!

Dr. Panush's patient suffered with typical arthritis symptoms, stiffness and swelling of her joints. These symptoms stopped when she ceased ingesting milk products. Dr. Panush tested her in a hospital under controlled conditions. He disguised foods so his patient did not know what she was eating and therefore could not be biased.

By this technique, Dr. Panush showed that his patient's observations about milk were correct. However, she believed two other foods aggravated her arthritis, too. A double blind test for these other two foods showed that she was wrong about the other two foods.

Discovering a patient whose arthritis was due to milk was an unexpected and fascinating observation. But, this doesn't mean *your* arthritis is due to milk allergy. In any situation where you or your doctors suspect food is responsible for a particular symptom, you must work *together* to prove beyond doubt that food is the causative factor. Dr. Panush practices in the arthritis clinic of a large teaching hospital in Florida where he sees many cases of arthritis each year. After he discovered that a food caused his patient's arthritis, he looked extra carefully for similar cases. Unfortunately, he and his colleagues have not found a similar case after three years of searching.

Helpful hint 1: Your doctors have to be open minded and listen to you when you tell them what you think is contributing to your symptoms.

Helpful hint 2: Of the hundreds of thousands of cases of arthritis in the United States, very few are due to milk allergy. So, don't stop your regular arthritis treatment on the slim chance that food allergy is the sole cause of your problem. Instead, consult your doctor and learn how to look into the possibility.

Migraine Headache Due To Food Allergy And An Entirely New Disease --Pseudo Food Allergy

Dr. Philip Fireman, from Pittsburgh, Pennsylvania, studied a patient who developed migraine headaches four hours after eating peanut, soy, corn, or beef. Several sophisticated x-ray tests (tomography and ultrasonography) confirmed his diagnosis. However, Dr. Fireman had just as difficult a time finding migraine patients who were allergic to foods as Dr. Panush had finding arthritis patients who were allergic to foods.

In fact, the problem of blaming various symptoms on food allergy when food allergy isn't at fault has created an entirely new disease called Pseudo Food Allergy. This was reported by Dr. Gordon Sussman of the University of Toronto. Pseudo Food Allergy is becoming widespread since many people are looking for easy answers to their medical problems and are quick to blame food allergy for various symptoms. Unwilling to take the trouble to be certain of their diagnosis, these people rely on skin and blood tests, even though these particular tests are known to be highly inaccurate and misleading when it comes to detecting food allergy.

Helpful Hint 1: There are many interesting individual case reports of people who suffer all kinds of symptoms due to food allergy. However, most of these cases are isolated. So, think twice before blaming food allergy for *your* symptoms just because you heard someone with similar symptoms had food allergy or because a skin or high-tech blood test says you have food allergy.

A Word About Avoidance Of Foods

When it comes to food allergy, avoidance is the best policy. However, you usually need to be an ace detective to avoid foods rigorously. Unfortunately, no matter how diligent you are, you can still make a mistake.

Dr. John Yunginger from Rochester, Minnesota, studied a case where a milk-allergic person ate a sorbet desert that was labeled kosher *and* milk free. Relying on the label, the sorbet seemed safe. However, just minutes after ingestion Dr. Yunginger's patient experienced hives and difficulty breathing. Upon chemical analysis of the sorbet, Dr. Yunginger found it contained milk protein contaminants.

Most of you are aware that labels and advertising cannot always be trusted. For food allergic individuals, this can be a matter of life and death.

Helpful hint 1: If you are allergic to foods, don't trust labels.

5

Allergy To Pets

Allergists have a reputation for disliking pets because they often tell their patients to get rid of their pets. On the other hand, patients sometimes have what seems to be an unreasonable attachment to pets that are making them sick as a dog.

Neither allergists nor patients are pig headed, though.

Both know the best treatment for allergy is avoidance. And, both know psychological studies show the companionship of a pet can be beneficial. So, in each case you and your health care professional must balance the good against the bad effect.

The first of the following four studies explains how pets cause allergy. The second proves that susceptible people can have symptoms in their homes even when they do not even own a pet. The third study shows how to wash your pet so your pet does not produce allergenic material. And the fourth study shows how to build your immunity to pets so they can't affect you even if you're exposed to them.

Cat Hair Doesn't Cause Allergy

Most of you have heard that cat hair causes allergy. This is not true.

Several doctors at the National Institutes of Health in Bethesda, Maryland, and a group of doctors who work in Germany proved it is not hair but a protein that is found in dander, saliva, and urine that causes allergy symptoms.

When they did the research, the doctors collected cat hair and removed the dander and dirt that was stuck to it. They rinsed off the saliva where the cats had licked themselves. Then, they exposed volunteer patients to dander, saliva, and cleaned hair.

The result? The volunteers reacted to dander and saliva. None of them reacted to the washed hair.

By the way, dogs and pet rodents like guinea pigs, hamsters, and mice are also allergenic because of a protein in their dander, saliva, and urine.

Helpful hint 1: If you're allergic to pets, you're allergic to a protein found in dander, saliva, and urine.

Helpful hint 2: Short-hair cats can produce as much dander as long-hair varieties. Therefore, they can cause just as much allergy.

No One Is Safe From Dogs And Cats

Doctors used to think if their patients weren't exposed to a pet, they couldn't blame pets for triggering symptoms.

Doctor B. Schwartz in Denmark proved this idea is wrong. She visited homes which had no pets and found that one third of the homes had measurable amounts of animal dander despite the absence of a pet. Furthermore, the dander was present in quantities that were sufficient to provoke symptoms in allergic patients.

Although no one really knows how animal dander got into these homes in the first place, Dr. Schwartz speculated that the dander was brought into the house by clinging to clothing when homeowners visited friends who owned pets.

Helpful hint 1: This study shows that avoidance of pets is often easier said than done.

Washing Cats Removes Allergenic Dander

Dr. H. J. Wedner of St. Louis, Missouri, performed a great service to cat lovers everywhere. In an experiment where he washed cats once a month in warm distilled water, Dr. Wedner reduced the amount of allergen by up to 50 percent after four washings. After nine washings, he reduced the allergen content by 75 percent.

Washing cats is not easy, but if you're dedicated to your cat and want to do some good for your allergies, this is a proven method.

Helpful hint 1: When it comes to animal allergy, avoidance is still the best policy

Helpful hint 2: No one has studied the effectiveness of washing birds and dogs, so you would have to do this on your own and see if it helps.

Helpful hint 3: If you stop washing your pet, the allergen returns. So, you must keep washing.

Helpful hint 4: If you're allergic to your pet and insist on keeping your pet, shower with a friend.

Allergy Injections For Cats And Dogs

For years many allergists offered no solution to pet allergy except avoidance. While this approach is guaranteed, there are other considerations. If you are like most people, you love your pet. Additionally, even if you gave up your pet, you are still exposed to your neighbors', friends', and relatives' pets.

Now, doctors are more willing to listen to you. And, instead of giving you an ultimatum, some are coming to the point of view that they can offer you the option to increase your immunity to animal allergens by using allergy injections. Although injections are time-consuming, they are effective. As long as your doctors raise the dose of serum to a high enough level, they can immunize you enough so that you can keep your pet without suffering symptoms.

One reason certain doctors were hesitant to recommend immunizing injections for pets was that they did not have access to the allergy literature and doubted that such injections would work. However, research has reconfirmed the usefulness of such injections. At a recent allergy meeting Dr. T. Van Metre presented a study in which *all* twenty-two patients he treated had significant relief with injections.

Each week Dr. Van Metre injected increasing doses of animal dander extract until he reached a maintenance level. At that point he continued injecting his patients once a month. This resulted in enough immunity so that pets could not trigger allergy symptoms.

But remember, the best treatment is still avoidance. Injections are only an alternative.

Helpful hint 1: If you are allergic to pets, the best treatment is avoidance.

Helpful hint 2: If you insist on having a pet, you can take allergy injections to build your immunity.

Helpful hint 3: If you choose to take allergy injections for pets, your dose of serum must be high enough to achieve a therapeutic effect. Otherwise, you're wasting your time.

6

Mold Allergy

Mold is the mildew or fungus which grows where it is damp, in places like bathrooms, near refrigerators, and around air conditioning units. Some varieties of mold grow where it is relatively dry. So, there isn't a universal rule about where you find mold.

Strictly speaking, you aren't allergic to mold. You're allergic to the spores that molds produce. These are microscopic pieces of mold that are released into the air, in the same way grasses, trees, and weeds release pollen grains.

The first study in this section shows that mold is not where you think it is. The second study explains an inexpensive and environmentally safe method to get rid of mold.

Mold Is In The Kitchen

Dr. Hector Busaniche from Santa Fe, Argentina, measured the mold levels in various rooms in eight homes. Fifty percent of the mold was in the kitchens due to moisture around refrigerators and sinks. Thirty percent was found in bedrooms, and 20 percent was in bathrooms. These findings were a surprise. Like most people, he had expected bathrooms to be the major source of mold.

When I ask my patients to remove mold, most of them deny they even have mold in their homes. They don't realize you cannot see mold with the naked eye unless there are thousands of colonies clumped together. Of those people who admit to mold in the home, like Dr. Busaniche, the first room they think of is their bathroom. This study shows that mold is everywhere.

Helpful hint 1: Mold is found throughout the home. But, the most common location for mold is the kitchen.

Heat Kills Mold

Dr. Jeff Miller, who practices allergy in Connecticut, studied a method of killing mold with heat. Although some molds can be heat resistant, the varieties Dr. Miller studied were 99 percent killed. He accomplished this by heating the air for about forty-eight hours. Of course, you've got to continue heating to prevent regrowth of mold, but heat is environmentally safe so this technique is without danger.

You can also use chemicals, called fungicides, to kill mold. These chemicals may be applied to ceilings, walls, floors, and even rugs. They can last for months at a time, depending on the type of chemical you use.

Helpful hint 1: If you use heat to kill molds, you must continue heating on a regular basis.

7

Allergy Testing

With any illness, you need to have a precise diagnosis to have the best chance for successful treatment. Without the correct diagnosis, treatment is merely guesswork.

After the history and physical examination, the most crucial information comes from the results of allergy testing. However, there is much misunderstanding about allergy testing because allergists perform so many different kinds of tests. There are scratch, intradermal, blood, provocation, sublingual, muscle, and diet tests. As you will read, some are useful, and some are not.

Although allergy testing can be simple and quick, it can also be made complex, costly, and time-consuming. The method utilized depends as much on a doctor's philosophy as on patients' expectations. Many doctors do not have time to study the various allergy tests and may not appreciate the benefits and disadvantages of each type. Patients, on the other hand, may believe they get what they pay for and think that more expensive tests must be more accurate.

In actual practice, you can be tested in fifteen minutes for every allergen imaginable. And, the results are available immediately.

The first of the following studies explains the grouping method. This technique reduces the total number of tests needed to investigate airborne allergens to a manageable

number. The second study explains how doctors concluded
that food allergy tests are only 19 percent accurate, no matter
what kind of test is utilized. The last study explains all you
need to know (and perhaps more than you want to know)
about three blood tests that are commonly used to diagnose
food allergy.

How To Reduce The Number Of Allergy Tests For Airborne Allergens
(Or, How To Cut The Cost Of An Allergy Workup)

Allergists don't want to make the mistake of overlooking
an allergen that might be contributing to your symptoms.
So, they commonly run 100, 150, or even 200 tests.
Although this will sound like a contradiction, doctors can
learn the same information from seventy-five tests as from
200 tests.

When it comes to airborne pollens such as grasses, trees,
and weeds, certain plants belong in families. So, if you are
allergic to one member of a family of plants, you are allergic
to the other members of the same family. For example, it is
unnecessary to test you for red, yellow, pink, and white
roses. A single test for the basic rose plant provides the same
information. People who are allergic to roses are not allergic
to the color. They are allergic to the plant itself.

There was recent proof of this from the laboratory of Dr.
Jean Bousquet in France. Dr. Bousquet showed that
members of the Oleacea family (olive, ash, privet, and
phillyrea) contain the same allergen. Thus, a person who is
allergic to olive is allergic to the other three species as well.

I have mixed emotions when I explain this grouping
method of testing. It's like having to apologize for being
practical. But, many patients equate the number of tests
their doctor performs to the thoroughness of their allergy

workup. They mistakenly believe that the more tests done the better their doctor.

Another way to reduce the number of tests is to omit tests for such things as camels and goats, unless, of course, you live with a camel or goat. The principle behind omitting tests for camels and goats is this: If you are not exposed to an allergen, the allergen cannot affect you no matter how allergic you are. To cite two practical examples, if you are highly allergic to kangaroos, you will never be bothered unless you live in a zoo. If you are fatally allergic to peanuts, you can't have symptoms unless you eat peanuts.

Helpful hint 1: It's rare that you require more than seventy-five scratch tests for a complete allergic analysis.

Helpful hint 2: An allergy workup is less costly and time consuming when fewer tests are done, yet the workup can still be thorough *if* the tests are chosen properly.

Inaccuracy Of Food Tests Confirmed

Food allergy is baffling to many people. Although there is no doubt that food allergy exists, there is a great deal of confusion over what types of problems food allergy can cause and how to investigate food allergy.

Two Types Of Hidden Food Allergy

There are two types of food allergy. One kind occurs within a few minutes after you eat a food. This is called an *immediate* reaction The other type is called *delayed* because it occurs *after* the food has been digested.

When you eat a food, your body converts the food into small by-products. As you know, this process is called digestion. People who react to unmetabolized foods are *immediate* reactors. People who react to metabolized foods are *delayed* reactors.

When a reaction occurs immediately you break out in hives, get itchy, or have a swollen face. This is a reaction to unmetabolized food. When your symptoms are delayed, the reaction is to the digested by-products of the food. Delayed reactions are responsible for numerous kinds of symptoms, such as headaches, asthma, fatigue, and nasal allergy, to name a few. For more details, see the appendix for the book *Hidden Food Allergy*.

Thus, there are two groups of people, immediate and delayed reactors. And, there are two kinds of causative agents, unmetabolized and metabolized foods.

The Problem With Blood And Skin Tests For Food Allergy

No laboratory in the United States sells digested foods for testing purposes. So, when skin or blood tests are performed for food allergy, doctors must use unmetabolized (undigested) foods. As you can imagine, tests using unmetabolized food would only uncover immediate-type food reactions. Yet the immediate reactions are the obvious ones. They begin soon after the food is ingested, so you know that something is wrong right away.

Delayed reactions which are due to metabolized by-products are difficult to pinpoint because they can occur from many hours to days later. And, as I said above, the tests in use today don't utilize digested by-products.

For years physicians knew that testing for foods was highly inaccurate, but recently, Dr. Charles Reed calculated exactly how inaccurate they are.

Dr. Reed performed skin and blood tests for food allergy on 102 people. He and his co-workers found thirty-one who showed reactions.

Then, Dr. Reed wanted to see if the tests had been accurate. To do this, he used a tried and true method. He fed the allergenic food, as indicated by the tests, to the subjects. This would tell him if those who had reacted on testing *also* reacted when they ate the food. This procedure is called a provocative challenge. Not wanting his subjects to be influenced by knowing what they were eating, Dr. Reed disguised the foods.

Of the thirty-one people who had positive tests, seven reacted upon eating the food. So, out of the thirty-one people who were supposed to be allergic, only seven actually had symptoms. This translated to an accuracy rate of 21 percent (7/31). This is not a good average! Twenty-one percent accuracy means 79 percent *inaccuracy*.

Helpful hint 1: Anyone who advocates relying on a test that is accurate only 21 percent of the time has got to be kidding! If you flip a coin, you get 50 percent accuracy.

Helpful hint 2: Anyone who lets themself be talked into doing a test that is accurate 21 percent of the time is desperate and grasping at straws.

Helpful hint 3: Twenty-one percent accuracy is true for the four skin tests, three blood tests, and the under-the-tongue (sublingual) tests that are still in use today, despite the dismal statistics.

Helpful hint 4: When it comes to subjecting patients to food tests, you can fool some of the people all of the time.

Three Blood Tests For Food Allergy

Blood tests for food allergy have become popular ever since scientists devised three basic methods of testing your blood for allergy. Sensing a high profit margin in such tests, commercial companies have rushed to create variations of the basic tests. As you might expect, each company claims its method is unique and best. At last count there were over eight variations on the market. And, the number increases every year.

Blood tests are the latest fad in allergy diagnosis. Their proponents claim the tests are faster and more accurate than skin tests. They also assert that using them spares you the supposed pain of the skin test procedure. Also, the blood tests sound more high-tech than skin tests.

As is true in many advertising situations, the proponents don't publicize the problems with their tests. Nevertheless, you should know the disadvantages. First, blood tests are slightly less accurate than skin tests. Your body's IgE is located in the skin surfaces of your nose, eyes, sinuses, lungs, and gastrointestinal tract. Only tiny amounts of IgE are found in your blood. Since allergic reactions occur on the surfaces of your body and not in your blood, testing your skin is more accurate than testing your blood.

Secondly, blood tests cost three to five times more than skin tests. So, if you undergo blood tests, you spend more money for slightly less accurate results.

As for the speed of the tests, skin tests take fifteen minutes. Blood tests need to be sent to a laboratory for processing. Then you need to wait for the report.

Because skin tests are more accurate, less costly, and show results immediately, trained allergists prefer skin tests.

The pain of skin testing is overdramatized and leads to groundless fear. Allergists don't dig huge needles into your skin. The scratch is superficial. There is not even bleeding.

The Three Kinds Of Blood Test

There are three kinds of blood test, called respectively the cytotoxic, histamine release, and RAST test.

Cytotoxic Test (Bryan's test, FICA test, Food Immune Complex Assay)

The cytotoxic test was proposed as a test for food and chemical allergies.

In the cytotoxic test, doctors extract your white blood cells and place them in little dishes. Then they add a food or chemical to each dish and observe whether your white cells break. If the cells break, you are said to be allergic to that food.

Regrettably, these tests have been proven highly inaccurate. The substances used for testing are *unmetabolized* instead of partially digested foods. Furthermore, many things can kill your white cells when they are removed from the protected environment of your body and placed in the dishes used in the cytotoxic testing procedure. If your white cells are simply incubated in these dishes, they die. And, breakdown of cells due to spontaneous death can easily be confused with breakdown upon addition of foods.

The cytotoxic test was developed in the early 1950s by Dr. Bryan (hence the original name Bryan's test). Thorough investigation has repeatedly shown the test is inconsistent. One day an unmetabolized food kills cells. Another day the same food does not kill the cells. Furthermore, this test does not take into account the effect of combinations of foods or whether a food is cooked, uncooked, pasteurized, frozen, or otherwise processed in a way that alters the food. There is no medical school, university laboratory, or licensed laboratory I know of in the United States that performs cytotoxic tests. Trained allergists don't do them. Only certain physicians do them in the privacy of their offices.

The claims that are made about the kinds of symptoms and diseases cytotoxic tests uncover are hard to believe. The list includes cancer, weight problems, emotions, headaches, arthritis, and gynecologic problems, to name a few.

> *If cytotoxic tests were helpful for half as many diseases as claimed, all your medical conditions would be due to allergy, and the only physician you would need throughout your life would be an allergist.*

Histamine Release Test

The histamine release test was proposed to investigate pollen and food allergy.

This test is similar to the cytotoxic test in the respect that doctors remove cells from your body and place them in small dishes. Then, they add foods and pollens to the dishes.

Instead of examining your cells for breakage, though, they measure the amount of histamine your cells release. Instead of examining your leukocyte-type white cells, as is done in cytotoxic testing, they examine basophil-type white cells.

The histamine test is accurate when used for pollens, but when used for foods, the test is as inaccurate as cytotoxic tests for the same reason--*unmetabolized* foods are used instead of metabolized by-products.

RAST Test

Finally there is the RAST family of tests. These have been proposed for detection of pollen and food allergy.

Several companies offer this type of test, but each company gives it a different name (FAST, PRIST, ELISA, MAST, RIST, STALLERZYM, CAP). Like the skin tests, they measure IgE antibody. However, measuring IgE in your blood costs three to five times more than measuring it in your skin.

For detecting airborne allergens, RAST-type tests are almost as accurate as skin tests. Thus, if you're investigating allergy to grasses, weeds, trees, and animal dander, if you do not mind spending three to five times more for blood tests, if the lower accuracy rate of RAST-type tests doesn't bother you, if you don't mind waiting a day to a week for the results, and if you don't mind having your blood drawn, RAST-type blood tests are acceptable.

However, for *food* allergy the RAST-type blood tests are as inaccurate as skin tests. They utilize *unmetabolized* foods instead of metabolized, digested by-products and produce results that are only 21 percent accurate.

If your auto mechanic told you he had an expensive test to find out if you need new brakes but 79 percent of the time the test was inaccurate, would you request the test? This is the situation with food allergy blood tests.

Some companies claim you ought to do blood tests for "clues" about food allergy. Put yourself in the shoes of someone who might be allergic to foods. Would you be willing to stop eating numerous foods for the rest of your life because someone had a clue based on a test that was 79 percent inaccurate? Or, would you want to know for sure?

The *Accurate* Food Allergy Test

My remarks may make you feel hopeless about the detection of food allergy. But, don't despair! There is a test that is 100 percent accurate. This test *always* works. It's cheap too! It's called an elimination diet. If you stop eating a food and get better and then eat the food and reproduce your symptoms, you have determined what foods to avoid. People groan when I mention elimination diets. But, you can't deny they are accurate.

Helpful hint 1: There are no new blood tests for allergy. There are only aggressive companies and doctors trying to market new versions of blood tests that are fifteen to thirty years old. By the time you read this book, you will undoubtedly hear of other "new" tests as marketing people become more inventive with new names for the old tests.

Helpful hint 2: Blood tests cost three to five times more than skin tests.

Helpful hint 3: Because airborne allergens do not have to be metabolized by the body into their allergenic form, both blood and skin tests *for airborne allergens* are accurate.

Helpful hint 4: Blood and skin tests for foods can lead to a common medical mistake which is to ignore *you* and treat your tests.

Helpful hint 5: To convince you to undergo costly blood testing, certain health professionals cast aspersions on skin tests. They say there can be delays in your reactions to a food, combinations of foods can cause your symptoms, skin tests are not accurate and elimination diets are tedious. These assertions imply that blood tests are the right approach.

In answer to these remarks, I agree there can be delay in onset of symptoms when food is ingested, food reactions can be due to combinations of foods, skin tests for foods are inaccurate, and elimination diets are tedious. But, and this is a big but, I have never read any textbook, scientific article, or magazine (and I've looked at as many as I could get my hands on) that showed blood tests are better. In fact, blood tests are worse! These doctors are so zealous and full of false hope they make you think that for a few dollars you can buy your answer without effort.

Helpful hint 6: If you insist on obtaining blood or skin tests to detect possible food allergies, you are looking for an easy way out. You are responding to advertising claims that reinforce what you want to hear instead of what is true.

Helpful hint 7: There is only one test that is 100 percent accurate for food allergy. That test is an elimination diet in which total abstinence from the food corrects the medical problem that bothers you. Even a double-blind food challenge test, where neither you nor your doctor know what you are eating, must be confirmed by eliminating a suspect food and determining whether your symptoms actually improved.

8

Allergy Injections

The phrase "allergy injection" has two different meanings. It can mean either an injection of a drug that temporarily alleviates your symptoms or an injection of an extract of allergenic substances that boosts your immunity. Unless you discuss which type of injection your health care professional is prescribing for you, you may not know whether you're receiving a short-term temporary or long-term permanent injection.

The first section of this chapter describes injectable drugs. The remaining sections deal with immunizing injections and cover such topics as the new polymerized serum that doctors hoped would allow patients to achieve permanent immunity with fifteen shots, how important it is for you to be religious about your injections, how to prevent allergy serum from deteriorating, how to improve your response when injections don't seem to be working, how doctors are experimenting with oral drops as a substitute for allergy injections, and finally, how to tell when you should stop taking allergy injections.

The One-Shot Cure For Allergies

Every so often a patient asks if I will give them the one shot that will cure their allergies. Usually they've heard about such an injection from a relative or friend.

There are many kinds of injections for allergy. And, each is used for a different purpose. Several injections are "one-shot". And, several are not. Below is a complete list of injections. If you hear about "one-shot", refer to the list and figure out whether it's the kind that would be appropriate for you.

Allergy shots can be divided into eight categories. Category five is the only one that contains natural substances which boost your immunity and thus counteract your excessive level of IgE antibody, which is the underlying cause of your allergy. The remaining seven categories are merely drugs which are supposed to relieve your symptoms--on a temporary basis.

1. Adrenaline or Epinephrine
   Adrenaline is prescribed to stop acute attacks of asthma or hives. Adrenaline injections last fifteen to twenty minutes. This is an old, old remedy that continues to be effective.

2. Sus-Phrine
   Sus-Phrine is a long-acting form of adrenaline. It lasts about eight to twelve hours and is prescribed for acute asthma or hives. Like adrenaline it has been available for a long time.

3. Albuterol
   Albuterol is a new adrenaline-like drug that lasts about thirty to sixty minutes longer than adrenaline. It's used for the same purpose as adrenaline, to stop acute attacks of asthma or hives.

4. Terbutaline
Terbutaline is another adrenaline-like drug that lasts about as long as adrenaline. In a few people it causes less stimulation of the heart and less jitteriness than adrenaline.

5. Allergy Immunizing Injections
Allergy immunizing injections contain no drugs. Instead, they contain natural substances like grasses, weeds, trees, dust, mold, and animal dander. They are given in gradually increasing quantity to force your body to make immunity.

Generally you need about twenty injections to build your dose to the point where you take the injections only once a month. After three years, you can usually stop. By then, most people have a kind of permanent immunity (see the section on Three Treatments of Allergy for details).

Immunizing injections are a standard treatment. They have been used for several decades with great safety in all ages and even during pregnancy. Their chief advantage is they attack your underlying problem and contain no drugs that could produce unwanted or deleterious side effects. The price you pay for trying to achieve a cure is that this treatment is definitely not "one-shot".

6. Antihistamines
Doctors give you an antihistamine injection when you have an acute allergic reaction such as after eating a food. Antihistamine injections work in your body for about four to six hours. The most commonly injected antihistamine is Benadryl (also called diphenhydramine).

7. Cortisone:

Cortisone, which is a steroid, is an anti-inflammatory drug. It relieves of all kinds of inflammation such as the inflammation due to arthritis, sports injuries, allergies, and third degree burns. Cortisone also kills certain kinds of cancer cells.

There are a many brands of cortisone, and they're sold in liquid, tablet, intravenous, ointment, and intramuscular preparations.

When a doctor gives you an intramuscular injection of cortisone, the drug can persist in your body up to three weeks. This will almost always stop your allergy symptoms. Cortisone won't build your immunity, but it sure feels good! If your allergy season is brief, this single shot will appear to have cured you. If your season lasts longer than three or four weeks, you may need several cortisone injections to carry you through. Of course next year your symptoms will return during your bad season and force you to take more cortisone. People tend to forget this. Instead they just remember cortisone stopped their symptoms and made them feel better.

Unfortunately cortisone can cause serious side effects like ulcer, weight gain, cataracts, and high blood pressure. These effects are dangerous. Unlike side effects of most drugs, the effects of cortisone may not go away even after you stop using it.

I suppose you could call cortisone an allergy shot, but I prefer to call it an injection of medicine which can stop symptoms for a period of time. When the cortisone wears off, you must take it again. Examples of brands of cortisone are Aristocort, Celestone, Decadron, Depo-Medrol, Dexamethasone, Kenalog, and Solu-Cortef.

8. Nasal Cortisone:
Nasal cortisone injections don't differ from other cortisone injections. I listed them separately because of the myth that when cortisone is injected into your nose it cannot produce side effects. No matter where or how cortisone is given to you, this drug is eventually absorbed into your body. Even when applied to your skin, cortisone is absorbed and can produce serious cortisone side effects.

Dr. Ray Slavin reported that the United States Food and Drug Administration has considered banning shots of nasal cortisone because several people have lost their vision. Losing your vision is a high price to pay to stop sneezing.

There are different brand names that disguise the fact that cortisone is a steroid. So, you may not know that you're getting cortisone unless you ask. The appendiz lists some of the brands to help you figure this out. Nevertheless, if you hear someone got a nasal injection for their allergy symptoms, you can be fairly certain they got cortisone.

I hope it's clear by now that cortisone, whether administered into your nose, muscle, or vein, is not a sure-fire, one-shot, quick cure. It can provide temporary relief up to three weeks at a time. And, this may feel like a cure. The problem is those darn side effects.

Helpful hint 1: There is no "one-shot" cure for allergy.

Helpful hint 2: There are two types of injections for allergy. One type contains various drugs that relieve your symptoms for a finite length of time. The other type are immunizing injections which contain no medicine. Instead immunizing injections build your immunity to the substances such as dust, pets, and pollen, that are responsible for your allergic reactions.

Helpful hint 3: Although you may not be told you are being given cortisone, a nasal injection that is said to be "one-shot for your allergies" strongly indicates you are getting cortisone.

New Type Of Allergy Injection Means Fewer Shots (Polymerized Extract)

Dr. Roy Patterson of Chicago spent many years attempting to improve allergy serum so that immunizing injections could be given less often and with greater safety.

For ragweed- and grass-allergic patients, Dr. Patterson developed a special serum called polymerized serum. Using this material, he gave twenty injections and produced permanent immunity in certain individuals.

Dr. Patterson accomplished this by altering molecules of ragweed and grass pollen. If you are not familiar with how allergy injections work, you'd have to understand the theory behind injection therapy in order to understand how Dr. Patterson succeeded with his special serum.

Ordinary allergy injections contain extracts of grasses, trees, weeds, dust, mold, and animal dander. These are the very substances to which you are allergic. There is no medication in them, no drugs of any kind.

Since you are allergic to the ingredients, the extract must be injected carefully or you might experience a reaction. To avoid reactions allergists raise the dose a little at a time. After approximately twenty build-up injections, which are given once or twice a week, patients reach a point that is called maintenance level. From then on, the injections are given every three to four weeks to maintain the immunity that has been achieved. At the end of three years, allergists try to stop treatment since, by then, most patients have permanent immunity. If you are asked to take injections longer than three years without even attempting to stop, this probably means your doctors are using the low- instead of the high-dose method for giving allergy shots.

The secret of Dr. Patterson's success was in finding a way to separate the allergy-provoking ability of allergens from their immune-stimulating ability. This enabled him to give larger doses of serum per injection without fear of an allergic reaction. It is similar to the feat scientists achieved when they separated the ability of polio, measles, and mumps viruses to infect the body from their ability to stimulate the body's immune system. Thus, when pediatricians vaccinate children, the children get better not worse, even though they are being injected with viruses that are ordinarily harmful.

With polymerized serum, Dr. Patterson was able to inject large amounts of pollen whose allergy-provoking potential had been blunted. Thus, each of his doses stimulated his patients to make huge quantities of antibodies without causing reactions. Previously, allergists needed to administer several injections of standard serum to achieve the same immunity as one injection of Dr. Patterson's serum. With more immunity per injection, patients not only went longer between injections, they achieved better results, too.

There are several disadvantages to these new injections, however. Dr. Patterson has not made polymerized serum for dog, cat, or mold. Therefore, if you are allergic to dog, cat, or mold, you would have to take traditional injections too.

This would actually *increase* the number of shots you'd need. Secondly, these substances haven't been used long enough to know if they're safe for a prolonged period of time. Traditional injections contain natural substances such as grasses, weeds, trees, and dog dander. These allergens enter your body every time you breathe. And, being natural, they are not inherently dangerous, unless you're allergic to them.

Polymerized serum is made with *altered* molecules, though. This makes them *unnatural*. And, only time will tell whether they are completely harmless. Finally, not everyone who took polymerized injections was completely cured after twenty shots. Most of the patients Dr. Patterson treated had to continue the injections just as do those who receive traditional allergy serum.

Helpful hint 1: Injections of polymerized serum are not really new. Dr. Roy Patterson's group and other groups have been studying them for almost fifteen years.

Helpful hint 2: There are several researchers who polymerize serum by a different technique from Dr. Patterson's. At the present time, no one is certain whose method is best.

Helpful hint 3: Those of you who are allergic to dust, pets, mold, and feathers would need injections of *traditional* serum for dust, pets, mold, and feathers *in addition* to polymerized serum for ragweed and grasses. Instead of reducing your visits and shots, this would actually increase the number of injections you'd need.

Helpful hint 4: Although there may be less risk of systemic reactions with polymerized sera, systemic reactions still occur. In the hands of people who've taken specialized allergy training, the systemic reaction rate using traditional sera is 0.45 percent. The statistics which have been published from Dr. Patterson's group using polymerized sera show a rate of 0.35 percent. Thus, although polymerized sera reduce the reaction rate, the reduction is only a slight improvement on what is already a well-controlled problem.

Helpful hint 5: No one knows the long term effects of injecting serum, such as polymerized serum, which contains altered proteins. Tests of immune function have shown no adverse effects from traditional extracts which contain natural proteins. But, polymerized extract has not been used by many people and must now enter the "consumer is guinea pig" stage. Doctors do not know for sure where this will lead.

Helpful hint 6: As with any new drug, treatment, or procedure there are pros and cons. Usually in such situations, the ultimate answer is that a certain segment of patients can be treated with polymerized serum successfully while others will need traditional serum. Always remember that a treatment that is helpful for *select* individuals is not necessarily helpful for *all* individuals.

New Polymerized Serum May Not Be Better Than Traditional Serum

Working in France, Dr. Jean Bousquet treated patients with a special polymerized serum and discovered that doses of 5,000 units of allergen produced the same immunity as 80,000 units. Interestingly, 5,000 units of allergen is the dose used by allergists who adhere to the high dose method that is recommended for immunization when utilizing standard, non-polymerized extracts.

So, if Dr. Bousquet's findings are confirmed, this means large doses of polymerized serum are not better than traditional serum. Of course, if you're not being treated with high doses of traditional allergy serum, you'd do better with the polymerized-type extracts.

Helpful hint 1: Although polymerized allergy serum seemed to be a great advance, preliminary information from Dr. Jean Bousquet's laboratory shows that super-high doses of polymerized serum produce no better results than the *recommended* doses of traditional serum.

Helpful hint 2: Those medical offices which routinely use low-dose injections ought to reconsider and begin reserving low doses only for those patients who cannot tolerate the recommended high doses.

Helpful hint 3: When you read about a new medical treatment, you must not automatically assume it is better.

Pollen Can Bother You After The Pollen Season Ends

At the end of your pollen season, you and your allergist have every reason to expect your symptoms to diminish as the pollen count drops. Unfortunately, your expectations are not always fulfilled. Several doctors in Minnesota found out why from studying patients who are allergic to red oak trees.

After the red oak season ended, the doctors discovered significant amounts of pollen on the ground. When the wind blew, this pollen became airborne and triggered symptoms in oak-allergic patients. Since this can happen with other pollens as well, you can see why you may feel ill after your season ends and why you may need to continue your treatment longer than you might have anticipated.

Helpful hint 1: Certain of you who have pollen allergies may have to continue allergy immunizing injections and allergy medication beyond your traditional pollinating season due to pollen that has blown to the ground during the active pollenating season and *recirculates* after the season is supposed to have ended.

Shots For Severe Asthma

Here's good news about a new shot for severe asthma attacks. Previously, if you were asthmatic, you sometimes had to rush to an emergency room for a shot of adrenaline (also called epinephrine) to stop an acute asthma attack. Although adrenaline works well, it doesn't last long. So, doctors often needed to give two or three shots in a row. As a side effect of this much adrenaline, some of you would become jittery, nauseous, or have a rapid pulse.

The new drug, called albuterol, belongs to the same category as adrenaline. But, by modifying the molecule, pharmacologists were able to reduce the side effects.

Dr. Sheldon Spector studied albuterol and found albuterol was an improvement over adrenaline for some people. For others, however, it was not.

Nevertheless, if you experience adrenaline side effects or if adrenaline doesn't work well for you, ask your doctor to try albuterol.

Strictly speaking, albuterol is not new. It has been available for a long time as a pill, liquid, and inhaler. However, using it as an injection is a new technique.

Helpful hint 1: In certain patients, albuterol lasts longer and has fewer side effects than adrenaline.

Helpful hint 2: Albuterol comes from the same parent drug as adrenaline.

Helpful hint 3: Other drugs in the adrenaline family are Alupent, Brethine, Bricanyl, Bronkometer, Ephedrine, Maxair, Metaprel, Primatene, Proventil, Salbutamol, Terbutaline, and Ventolin.

Discovery That Allergy Serum Loses Potency Quickly

Allergy serum loses its strength when it is exposed to warm temperatures. This is called *thermal* decay. To prevent this from happening, allergists store your serum in a refrigerator. Even at refrigerator temperatures, though, your serum can lose its potency with the passage of time due to *spontaneous* decay.

Dr. Harold Nelson studied the decay phenomenon and found that over the course of several months bottles of sera are removed from the refrigerator many times in order to prepare injections for each appointment. Thus, each bottle of serum undergoes many days of warming and can become unacceptably weak.

This is a serious problem because the weaker the serum the less immunity it can stimulate and the less effective are allergy shots.

The most commonly used sera are the aqueous or watery type, even though these are subject to the fastest deterioration. The slowest to lose strength are glycerin- and albumin-based. Although doctors have known that aqueous are the most susceptible to decay, many medical offices ignore this and continue to use the aqueous solution because the glycerinated kind can sting you for a moment.

My teachers, Drs. William Deamer and Lee Frick, insisted that glycerin be used because this kind of serum retains its potency best. Furthermore, despite the *theoretical* possibility of stinging, very few patients actually have problems. Thus, it does not make sense to use weaker and less effective solutions when the vast majority of people tolerate the strong and active material.

In addition to sera that deteriorate quickly, there is a serum that is actually weak from the start. This is the situation with a serum called Allpyral. Allpyral is made by a unique process. And, many years ago Dr. Larry Lichtenstein at Johns Hopkins Medical School showed that this process weakens the ingredients so that they don't stimulate immunity as strongly as the standard extracts that most companies make.

However, Allpyral is of inestimable help for super-sensitive patients who cannot tolerate standard allergy extracts. But, the majority of you are not super-sensitive. And, doctors who prescribe Allpyral exclusively are treating all their patients with less than the full immunizing doses which their patients might be capable of tolerating.

Helpful hint 1: It's better to have burning and stinging for a few minutes than to take injections that don't burn or sting but are so weak they don't do much good.

Helpful hint 2: The stronger the serum injected, the more immunity you make. The more immunity you make, the longer you can go between injections and the fewer doctor visits you'll need.

Helpful hint 3: You can tell your doctor that you'd prefer strong serum and you're willing to put up with a little burning in order to take advantage of the benefits of strong allergy serum. Besides, despite the talk of burning and stinging, most people tolerate strong injections without difficulty.

Dust Mite In Your Allergy Serum Can Ruin Your Chance For Successful Immunization

Ordinarily, allergists make a personalized mixture of allergy serum based on your particular test results. This recognizes that you are a unique individual. However, due to a large volume of patients, certain medical offices and clinics prescribe the generic mixtures for everyone. This latter method is easier than making and storing special bottles for each patient. But, the custom assumes everyone is sensitive to the identical substances to the same degree. As you probably know, everyone's allergies are *different*. Nevertheless, many people obtain satisfactory relief from generic mixtures.

When allergists treat you with mixtures, whether personalized or generic, they sometimes include house dust mite in your preparation. Dr. S. Kagan has discovered that certain enzymes found in dust mite attack and weaken other allergens such as grasses, trees, and weeds. Weaker serum would, of course, reduce the level of immunity your body can attain.

There are several ways to avoid this problem: keep serum cold, use glycerin extract, and maintain separate bottles for dust mite injections.

Helpful hint 1: Mixing allergens may seem simple. But, like many aspects of allergy, there are pitfalls that need to be avoided.

New Reason Found For Injection Failure In Ragweed Allergy

Ragweed is one of the most bothersome and allergenic plants in the United States. Its pollen affects people wherever it is found. Fortunately for us on the West Coast, there is very little ragweed. East of the Rocky Mountains, though, ragweed is a major allergy problem.

Ragweed produces so much pollen that the number of grains can be easily counted. So, during ragweed season, radio stations in the East and Midwest report the pollen count beginning from the middle of August until early October. If you suffer from ragweed allergy, these reports tell you how sick you should be just in case you don't already know it.

Dr. John Santilli noticed that some of his ragweed-sensitive patients did not feel better after taking allergy injections. Upon investigation, he discovered that these patients were allergic to molds which are found in high concentration at the same time of year ragweed is in the air. Unfortunately, molds had not been included in these patients' serum. This made their treatment incomplete.

Only when your doctors search for *all* possibilities and treat you for *all* your sensitivities will you obtain optimum relief.

Helpful hint 1: Even if you have a classic history for a particular allergy, your doctors should check all possibilities by thorough testing before they finalize your treatment.

Helpful hint 2: If you have ragweed allergy and are not obtaining satisfactory relief, ask your doctor to reevaluate you. You may be one of those who has mold allergy, too.

Oral Drops Might Replace Allergy Injections

Dr. Ebbe Taudorf, who does research in Denmark, tried to immunize patients without injections. His idea was to dissolve pollen in a special solution and administer this in gradually increasing quantities to allergic individuals. Other physicians had tried a similar approach but had not succeeded.

In Dr. Taudorf's hands, patients achieved partial immunity against allergic reactions to various weeds. Unfortunately, they had no relief for their allergy to grasses. Another disappointment was that the oral drops helped eye symptoms but did not improve nasal symptoms.

Furthermore the drops were not innocuous. Many patients suffered from diarrhea and abdominal pain due to gastrointestinal allergic reactions to the ingested allergens.

Dr. Taudorf plans to experiment with different doses of drops and even with tablets to see if he can increase the beneficial effect and minimize the undesirable effects. So far, though, he has not found the answer.

Helpful hint 1: Physicians are searching for a reliable technique to replace allergy injections. So far, they haven't figured out a foolproof method.

Helpful hint 2: If you suffer from allergy to airborne pollens and are waiting for an easy cure, you should probably obtain treatment now instead of waiting for a medical breakthrough that may never come to pass.

How Often To Repeat The Skin Tests

Should your skin tests be performed once in a lifetime or once a year? Is it useful to do them at the end of a series of allergy injections or in the middle?

Dr. T. Coleman studied these questions. From his investigations, he concluded that you need skin tests initially to diagnose your allergic problem. But, you rarely need to repeat the tests.

Your allergies do not vary from day to day, week to week, month to month, or even from year to year. Over several years your sensitivities might change, but, generally speaking, there won't be earthshaking changes.

Additionally, Dr. Coleman's studies confirmed what allergists had known for many years: The results of scratch tests won't determine when you are ready to stop allergy injections.

You would think that retesting would help your doctors decide the appropriate time to stop allergy injections. After all, when you've completed several years of injections it's only logical to suppose that skin tests would show you have built your immunity to the point where you can discontinue your treatment.

Unfortunately, the body doesn't work that way. Although studies show your immunity *increases* and your sensitivity *decreases* after a series of injections, this doesn't indicate that you can stop your shots. It doesn't indicate you need to continue them either.

Dr. Coleman divided his patients into two groups: a group where symptoms *did not* return upon discontinuing shots and a group where symptoms *did* return upon discontinuing shots.

After carefully reviewing the medical records of both groups, Dr Coleman could not find how to predict who would be successful stopping shots. Not even blood or skin tests told him the answer. Thus, he concluded there was only one way to find out whether a patient could stop injections without relapsing. A patient had to stop and observe what their body would do.

If you've used the high dose therapy, you may usually try stopping treatment after three years of monthly injections. If you use the low dose method, you must usually continue your shots longer.

The reason allergy tests aren't useful at predicting the outcome is that they indicate your level of immunity *at the time the tests are performed*. What you want to know, though, is what your immunity will be after you stop the shots. Will it stay high or drop off? Will it drop slowly or quickly? As you are aware, you need a crystal ball to predict anything, *including* what will happen if you stop allergy injections. At the present time, no one is making good crystal balls.

Are there situations where it is appropriate to be retested? Yes. If you develop a sudden change in your symptoms, if many years (five to ten) have elapsed since your initial tests were performed, or if you move to an area which has *significantly* different allergens from where you were first tested, you may need to be retested.

Helpful hint 1: There is no particular benefit in automatically repeating your skin or blood tests every year.

Helpful hint 2: Skin and blood tests do not indicate when you can stop allergy immunizing injections without worrying about a relapse.

Helpful hint 3: Three situations where it is useful to retest for allergy sensitivities are: if many years have passed, if you have moved to an area with significantly different allergens, or if your pattern of symptoms has changed.

9

Medications Which Alleviate Allergy

If I asked you to tell me the first way you tried to control your allergy symptoms, you'd probably say, "I took some medication." Although drugs are usually the initial treatment for allergy, they are poorly understood and often incorrectly used.

Allergy medication can be purchased with or without a prescription. As you know from being bombarded with advertising, there are tablets, capsules, liquids, sprays, injections, and inhalants. According to manufacturers' claims, these products work flawlessly. In many cases the drugs perform up to the claims that are made. However, in many cases they do not. None of the companies are so sure of their products that they give you a written guarantee.

The following studies describe how the newer drugs work, how they help, how to use them properly, and what kinds of side effects you should watch for.

The first study explains how antihistamines might make your asthma worse. The next two studies tell about an antihistamine that was advertised as not making people sleepy. The fourth describes an antihistamine that can last all day. The fifth one tells about the six kinds of adverse reactions that drugs can cause. Then there is a report that theophylline can produce jitteriness in children.

Next is a warning about breaking asthma medication pills in half, two exciting new drugs for asthma, and a report that tells you about a problem that can arise when you mix various types of medication. Finally, there is a warning about a blood pressure medication that can make your allergies worse.

Antihistamines Can Make Asthma Worse

Because antihistamines are known for drying mucus, physicians were hesitant to recommend them to asthma patients for fear that the antihistamines would dry the mucus in the lungs. This would make it more difficult to breathe. There are warnings about this in nearly all medical textbooks.

Years ago, though, allergists reviewed the original research and discovered the studies had not been done carefully. So, despite the dire warnings, allergists prescribed antihistamines for patients who had runny noses even if the patient also had asthma. Over the years the allergists were proven correct. Asthmatics did not go into fits of coughing or stop breathing upon using antihistamines. Thus, those individuals who had nasal symptoms didn't have to suffer just because they had asthma, too.

Just when all the allergists were comfortable prescribing antihistamines for asthmatics, Dr. Diane Schuller discovered a group of children whose asthma got worse when they took antihistamines, thus confirming the original fears.

Did this mean that allergists were wrong and textbooks were right? No. Dr. Schuller had merely found a small *subgroup* of children who became worse. Even in her studies the majority of patients tolerated antihistamines without ill effects. Furthermore, adverse reactions only occurred with certain antihistamines. So, when one antihistamine created a problem she simply switched her patients to another.

Helpful hint 1: If you use an antihistamine and your asthma flares up, throw the antihistamine into the garbage can.

Helpful hint 2: If you have a stuffy nose, try an antihistamine. You have a 98 percent chance it will help you without making your asthma worse.

New Antihistamine Doesn't Make You Sleepy

Have you heard or read of an antihistamine that doesn't make you sleepy? If not, you will. Drug companies are continually searching for new chemicals. What they've discovered so far is the subject of this section.

According to the technical definition of an antihistamine, cimetadine (brand name Tagamet) is an honest-to-goodness antihistamine. However, Tagamet belongs to a completely different category of antihistamine from the ones that help allergies.

Tagamet is an anti-ulcer medicine which works by stopping your stomach from producing acid. Because Tagamet is so effective, it is spawning a family of antihistamines that have no drowsy side effects. However, except in very rare circumstances such as in certain cases of hives, Tagamet, and the other members of that family of drugs (Ranitidine, Zantac, Pepcid), will not help allergies.

This is a case where the facts are more complicated than they might appear. You see, there are two kinds of antihistamines, called H1 and H2. The H1 kind helps allergy symptoms such as sneezing, nasal stuffiness, itchy eyes, runny nose, postnasal drainage, and hives. The H2 kind reduces acid in the stomach. The H1 kind can make you drowsy. The H2 kind will not. Thus, if you take Tagamet, you won't be sleepy, but you won't have much relief of your allergies either.

How To Find An Antihistamine
That Works For Your Allergies

Let's say you need an H1 type of antihistamine for your allergies. Could you find one that doesn't make you sleepy? Is there a systematic way to go about it? H1 antihistamines have such a terrible reputation it might seem hopeless to even try.

Luckily there is a way to find such a drug. Thanks in part to work done by Dr. Guy Settipane, doctors have an understanding of H1 antihistamines that makes it easy to figure out which is best for a particular individual.

First, if you read about a new drug that doesn't produce drowsiness, be skeptical. There are really *no* new H1 antihistamines. There are over 103 brands of antihistamines. And, they can be grouped into four basic categories. Clever manufacturers change the shape, color, and name of these drugs. They make tablets which last four hours and twelve hours. They add decongestants and aspirin to create another brand of the same drug. But, despite these modifications there are still only *four* categories of antihistamine.

Some categories work for some people, and others work for others. The way to find the best brand for *you* is to try them all. Each of your bodies is different. You have different weight, height, muscle, fat, and metabolism. You handle medications differently. No one can predict how you will react to an antihistamine, or any other kind of drug.

Experimenting with over one hundred drugs sounds like a lot of work. But you can do it in four days. Yes! You read correctly -- four days.

Use one representative of each of the four categories. That is the way to *systematically* find the one that's best for you. The technique is explained in *Take Charge of Your Health.*

Back to the drowsy issue! When Dr. Settipane tested for the drowsy effect, he found up to 15 percent of people became drowsy when they used H1 antihistamines. The rest did not. So, most of you can take *any* antihistamine without a problem. Others will have to experiment a little to find a suitable one. For those that cannot find an H1 antihistamine, there are other types of medicine that can help you.

I don't want to belabor the point, but don't automatically jump to the conclusion that you cannot take antihistamines even if you've had bad luck with several different ones. You may merely have been taking the same drug under a different brand name.

Some doctors may disagree and say there are more than four categories. They might give you a few other drugs. Don't quibble. Chemists disagree about this. Humor your doctor and be willing to try a few extra pills. But if your health care professionals recommend *ten* different antihistamines, they are teasing you.

Ninety-five percent of over-the-counter drugs contain the identical category of antihistamine. Benadryl is the exception. It comes from a category different from the others.

You may be interested in the names of the four categories. They are ethanolamines, alkylamines, ethylenediamines, and the last category is composed of ring structures. These are technical names. You will not find them on labels. Even many doctors will not be familiar with them.

Helpful hint 1: H1 antihistamines alleviate allergy symptoms, but they can cause drowsiness in about 15 percent of people.

Helpful hint 2: The way for each of you to find the most effective antihistamine with the fewest side effects is to try a representative of each of the four categories.

Helpful hint 3: Antihistamines don't cure anybody of anything. They are for symptomatic relief. So, take the least amount that controls your symptoms.

The Newest New Antihistamine That Doesn't Make You Sleepy

Marion Merrell Dow Company developed an antihistamine that newspaper and magazine headlines proclaim won't make you drowsy. The drug is said to "separate sedation from relief." This is a typical example of how you must be careful when you hear a medical claim.

The drug is called Seldane, or Terfenadine. Unfortunately, Seldane is not a panacea. Some people find it helps, and some do not. Some find it makes them sleepy, and some do not. In this respect Seldane is similar to all the drugs that doctors have been using for years.

What led newspapers to headline the non-drowsy effect is a common reaction of newspaper and magazine editors. They isolate one fact and emphasize what is newsworthy, not what is necessarily a balanced appraisal.

When Seldane is compared to an antihistamine called Chlorpheniramine, Seldane causes less drowsiness in certain individuals. However, the company did not compare Seldane to each of the other categories of antihistamine. Limiting a comparison to one possibility out of a number of possibilities is a tried and true method to make a product seem favorable. For example, if you compare Hawaiian to Korean apples, the Hawaiian apples may taste terrific. But if you compare Hawaiian to Washington state apples, you would find Washington apples were head and shoulders above the rest.

Another aspect that newspaper editors failed to mention, but which the drug company was honest about, was that Seldane caused more weakness, dry mouth, and appetite increase than several other antihistamines.

Thus, Seldane is an excellent drug and is definitely worth trying. But, Seldane is not a miracle.

There is another factor to consider when you hear about a new drug. You must ascertain whether the drug helps you. If a drug's only redeeming value is that it does not make you sleepy, it will not be of much use.

Like all drugs, Seldane has a good effect in some, a bad effect in some, and no effect in some.

Helpful hint 1: Newspaper articles tend to emphasize what editors hope will sell their papers. They do not necessarily give a balanced view.

Helpful hint 2: The only way to learn whether an antihistamine will help you is to try the antihistamine.

Helpful hint 3: The only way for you to learn whether an antihistamine will cause side effects is to try it.

Helpful hint 4: There is no perfect antihistamine that suits everyone. Each of you has a different metabolism.

Helpful hint 5: If an antihistamine does not make you sleepy but does not relieve your symptoms, you accomplish nothing when you take it.

A Twenty-Four Hour Antihistamine

Every year at the meeting of the American Academy of Allergy and Immunology the latest research and newest antihistamine compounds are discussed. Some of the drugs are variations of medications that have already been approved for use. Some are so new they don't even have a name, merely a research number that identifies them. Some hold great promise, and some do not.

Astemizole (brand name Hismanal) is an antihistamine that showed exceptional promise.

This drug, which was used in Europe, Canada and Mexico for many years, had a lower rate of producing side effects than other antihistamines. But, its major advantage was that it lasted twenty-four hours in most individuals. Taking a pill once a day makes it easier to comply with the instructions.

As with many drugs there is a trade-off when using Hismanal. This drug often takes three days to begin working. Many doctors don't explain this to their patients. If you are used to and want instant relief, you will probably not be happy with Hismanal.

Helpful hint 1: Once in a while truly new drugs are developed. Hismanal is not really one of the *truly* new drugs.

Helpful hint 2: Astemizole, like other antihistamines, is useful only for symptomatic relief. When it is prescribed, you must usually take it three days before it begins working.

Six Kinds Of Adverse Reactions To Drugs

When the question of drug reactions comes up, it's tempting to take a shortcut and blame allergy without giving any thought to the situation. However, you and your doctors must go through the list of the various kinds of reactions systematically and carefully. Otherwise you may get the wrong diagnosis. This kind of mistake will usually lead to incorrect treatment. There are six kinds of drug reactions you need to consider.

1. Overdose

Overdose is a reaction due to taking an excess amount of medicine or because your body accumulates too much of a drug. A child who swallows too much aspirin is an example of taking excess medicine. A person who has depressed liver or kidney function and therefore cannot dispose of drugs properly is an example of the other way you can be subject to overdose.

2. Intolerance

Intolerance is a normal effect of a drug which is exaggerated in some individuals. For example, aspirin can cause mild irritation of the lining of your stomach. Under ordinary circumstances you won't notice this. However, certain individuals are *so* sensitive they get an ulcer and vomit when taking aspirin.

3. Idiosyncrasy

Idiosyncrasy is a reaction that occurs in specific susceptible individuals. When certain individuals use Thorazine, which is a relaxant, their muscles go into temporary spasm and their body twists like a pretzel.

4. Side effects

Side effects are undesirable but sometimes unavoidable responses to a drug. Decongestants and bronchodilators come from a category of drug called sympathomimetics. These open your nose and the airways in your lungs. However, both of them can increase your heart rate and make you jittery at the same time they are opening your respiratory passages.

5. Secondary effect

Secondary effects are indirect. Antibiotics kill bacteria that cause infection. However, they can also kill *beneficial* bacteria that reside in your intestine. This can lead to overgrowth of *harmful* bacteria, a condition which can reuslt in diarrhea and even a fungus infection called candida or monilia.

6. Allergy

Allergic reactions occur from an immune response. This has nothing to do with the pharmacologic action of the drug. Allergy is due to your body having made an excessive amount of IgE antibody which reacts with the drug and causes itching, hives, asthma, or collapse.

Helpful hint 1: Most drug reactions are *not* allergic.

Helpful hint 2: If you experience anything different from usual when you take a drug, consult your doctor to find out if you are having an adverse reaction to the drug and *what kind* of adverse reaction it is.

How Vitamin C Was Thought To Help Allergies

You've probably heard many miraculous claims for vitamin C. Those who support vitamin C's virtues say it can prevent various diseases like colds, cancer, and allergies. When claims seem too good to be true, scientists endeavor to separate the facts from the fancy.

One such investigator was Dr. Harold Nelson. He studied the effect of vitamin C on allergies. Curiously, there's a relationship between vitamin C and histamine. Vitamin C lowers the level of histamine in the bloodstream. Of course there is not that much histamine in your bloodstream to begin with. Most of the histamine in your body is contained within certain cells. Nevertheless, if histamine was in your bloodstream, vitamin C could reduce its level.

Dr. Nelson fed volunteers vitamin C and measured their allergy symptoms. He also tested their skin sensitivity before and after they ingested vitamin C. Despite ingesting 2,000 milligrams of vitamin C a day, the skin tests and symptoms did not change. The only thing vitamin C achieved was a reduction in the blood level of histamine.

As you read previously, *many* chemical mediators contribute to the allergic reaction. So, even though vitamin C can reduce your blood level of histamine, this would only reduce *one* of the multiple chemical mediators that cause allergic reactions.

Helpful hint 1: When you hear a scientist advocate that a complex disease like allergy can be treated by a single vitamin, you must make a superhuman effort not to be seduced by the simplicity of the proposal.

Helpful hint 2: Although vitamin C can affect histamine levels in your bloodstream, it doesn't have any effect on your allergy symptoms or skin tests.

Helpful hint 3: Allergy sufferers have had a lot of disappointments over the years from eager salespeople who've claimed they had discovered a miracle cure.

Theophylline Can Cause Emotional Problems In Children

Theophylline is one of the most common drugs used to treat asthma. It has relatively few side effects and works well. However (doesn't there always seem to be a "however" in medicine) excess theophylline can create symptoms such as nausea, headaches, jitteriness, and an abnormal heartbeat. The most common reasons for excess theophylline are:

1. too high dose
2. taking Tagamet (cimetadine) while using theophylline
3. smoking
4. using erythromycin
5. a viral infection

In addition to the overt adverse effects of theophylline, doctors have discovered *subtle* side effects. A physician in Seattle, Dr. Clifton Furukawa, found that theophylline can be responsible for behavioral and learning problems in children. This applies only to particular children. So, if you notice a change in your child's behavior, problems with sleep, or the onset of a learning disability, *or* if teachers have noticed such changes, consult your doctor. Most behavioral and learning disorders are *not* due to this drug, but it's worth considering. When theophylline causes these symptoms, the treatment is simple: adjust the dose of the drug. Then, the problem will cease.

Helpful hint 1: When you take a medication and notice a change in the way you feel, act or behave, consult your doctor to see if the change might be due to the drug.

Tests For Theophylline Drug Level And Why The Tests Are Frequently Unnecessary

When treating asthma with theophylline, most allergists aim to keep the blood level between ten and twenty micrograms. To measure the level, allergists used to have to send a sample of your blood to an outside laboratory.

Now there are tests that enable your doctors to perform the measurement in their office. This makes it easier to keep track of the efficacy of your asthma treatment. In some offices the blood level is measured at every visit. Then, the dose is changed until the target level is achieved.

Dr. Charles Reed examined the practice of frequent testing. He concluded it is unnecessary to test everyone *routinely*. Several studies have shown that low to moderate doses of theophylline (even below ten micrograms) are sufficient to control asthma in most people. So, there is no need to routinely put *all* of you on high doses and subject you to possible side effects.

Dr. Reed, who works at the Mayo Clinic, went so far as to say that only the *severest* cases of asthma must be given high doses which are close to toxic levels and which require frequent monitoring of your blood.

Helpful hint 1: If you take theophylline and feel side effects, ask your doctor to test you to determine whether you are taking too much.

Helpful hint 2: Theophylline blood levels don't have to be done routinely. The major exception is when you must be hospitalized for a severe attack.

Helpful hint 3: It's not wrong for your doctors to perform *routine* testing for theophylline, but don't be overly impressed that they are practicing advanced medicine. In most cases, routine testing is not necessary.

Helpful hint 4: There are certain drugs and several illnesses that can raise or lower the theophylline level. Respectively, this can create toxic effects from too much or render theophylline ineffective from too little.

Decrease Theophylline Level	Raise Theophylline Level
1. young children	1. Tagamet
2. smoking	2. liver disease
3. high protein diet	3. erythromycin
4. phenobarbital	4. viral infection
5. phenytoin	5. heart failure
	6. pneumonia

Breaking Asthma Tablets To Obtain Half-Doses Can Be Dangerous

Doctors generally prescribe your dose of asthma pills based on your body size. The dose also depends on the severity of your symptoms, which, as you probably know from your own experience, will vary depending on the degree of your exposure, the season of the year, and what other allergens you had contact with that day. Thus, for a variety of reasons, your doctor may tell you to break your allergy tablets in half to increase or decrease your dose.

Dr. Cheryl Lutz discovered you cannot count on obtaining the correct dose when you break the 100 mg size of a pill called Theo-Dur. The tablet is scored, indicating that it is designed to be broken in half. But when Dr. Lutz measured the blood levels of theophylline, which is the active ingredient in Theo-Dur, the halves produced unequal results. The half tablet was absorbed faster than the whole one. Thus the time to reach maximum blood level varied and resulted in less control of symptoms and greater tendency to experience side effects in certain patients.

Helpful hint 1: If you notice unusual responses when you use a half-tablet or half-capsule of medication, consult your doctor.

Albuterol Powder And Ketotifen--Two New Drugs For Asthma

Albuterol powder and Ketotifen tablets are two new and exciting asthma drugs.

1. Albuterol Powder

Albuterol was first sold as a liquid in a squeeze bottle. When having an asthma attack, you had to squirt the medicine into your lungs. *Powdered* albuterol is a new idea. The brand name is Rotocaps. You may wonder why doctors are excited about a powder that comes in a capsule when the liquid is already available.

Liquid albuterol in pressurized cannisters is difficult to use. When you activate the cannister, you must inhale at precisely the right moment. Otherwise, the drug does not penetrate deep into your lungs. The timing is tricky, especially if you are having difficulty breathing. Picture yourself gasping for breath and trying to inhale deeply at the same time.

At a recent scientific meeting of the American Academy of Allergy, Dr. James Kemp explained how albuterol powder works. When you need medication, you place a capsule in a small container and twist the container, thereby breaking the capsule and spilling the powder into the bottom of the container. Then you suck the powder into your lungs. The result is effective and widespread distribution of the drug onto the surface of your lungs.

2. Ketotifen

Ketotifen is a drug which, like cromolyn, can *prevent* allergy reactions. Since cromolyn is not absorbed by your body, you must spray it into your eyes, nose, lungs, or all three locations, depending on what type of symptoms you have. Wouldn't it be nice to take a pill that could travel to *all* parts of your body and do the work of three sprays?

Ketotifen may achieve this. The drug seems to work as does cromolyn to *prevent* allergy symptoms. And, since Ketotifen is absorbed, one pill can actually do the job of three sprays.

As with any drugs, Albuterol Powder and Ketotifen tablets help certain individuals and do not help others.

Helpful hint 1: Sometimes a drug is "new" simply because doctors learn more efficient and more effective ways to deliver them to affected parts of your body.

Helpful hint 2: No matter why a drug is new, each person must determine, for themselves, whether the drug alleviates their symptoms.

Vomiting And Nausea From Allergy Medicines

This is a classic example of how drugs can react with each other and make you ill. It's a good reminder to be careful when mixing medications.

Cephalosporins are antibiotics which are related to penicillin. Since they don't cause as many allergic reactions as penicillin, they're safer to use. From the time of their inception, the drug industry has improved them by creating newer, stronger, and more stable compounds. We are now into what is called the third generation of cephalosporins.

Four of the new cephalosporins can create a special problem for allergy sufferers. When your body metabolizes these four (see below), it breaks them into pieces, one of which happens to be disulfiram or Antabuse. You may have heard of Antabuse. This drug is prescribed to prevent alcoholics from drinking. When taken with alcohol, Antabuse produces flushing, throbbing headaches, vomiting, chest pain, weakness, and confusion. This is a forceful deterrent to those who drink.

Unfortunately, many liquid allergy preparations, such as antihistamines, cold remedies, and theophyllines, contain up to 12 percent alcohol. Thus, if you are taking any of the four cephalosporins, you will have Antabuse in your bloodstream as the cephalosporin is metabolized. If at the same time you use a preparation containing alcohol, you will experience the alcohol-Antabuse reaction. This is not fun.

The four cephalosporins are cefamandole (Mandol), cefoperazone (Cefobid), cefuroxime (Zinacef, Kefurox), and moxalactan (Moxam). There will undoubtedly be more brands of third generation cephalosporins as drug companies do more research, so consult your doctor.

Helpful hint 1: Mixing drugs is not a good idea unless you know what you're doing.

Helpful hint 2: Certain cephalosporins are broken down to an Antabuse-like chemical.

Beta Blockers Can Make Asthma Worse

Over the past few years beta blockers have been prescribed to treat conditions such as angina, hypertension, glaucoma, and even migraine headache. Common beta blockers are Inderal, Corgard, Blocadren, Lopressor, Tenormin, and Timoptic.

In certain individuals beta blockers are a two-edged sword. Although effective for cardiac and vascular conditions, they can increase allergic symptoms.

Dr. John Toogood from Canada reported that patients who take beta blockers can suffer heightened allergic reactions to foods, certain drugs, insect stings, and X-ray contrast material. Although allergy injections do not contain drugs, beta blockers can increase your reactions to allergy injections as well.

These findings do not mean you must stop using beta blockers. They merely mean you must be alert to the possibility that this drug can backfire. So, be prepared to switch to another type of drug if you experience adverse effects when a doctor prescribes a beta blocker for you.

Helpful hint 1: If you're using drugs and notice new or different symptoms, consider the possibility that the drugs are responsible for the change in your condition. And, consult your doctor.

10

Nasal Sprays

According to the National Institutes of Allergy in Bethesda, Maryland, over nineteen million people in the United States suffer from nasal allergy symptoms. Since nasal sprays are efficient and convenient, many of you may have tried them at one time or another. Their chief advantage is they deliver medication directly to your nasal membrane where you need it most.

The following is a summary of the types of nasal sprays that are available, how they work, and what side effects can occur. Some of the sprays are relatively new. Others have been around for years.

Nasal Sprays For Allergy

There are old and new nasal sprays. But, the nasal spray story is so complex it's best to describe old and new together.

The situation is similar to antihistamines. Some sprays are "new" because the manufacturer devised a new package for the same old ingredient. Some are "new" because they are new to the United States. In other words, there is nothing revolutionary. Remember, "new" can mean different things to different people.

1. Salt water

Salt water is a tried and true "drug" for relieving nasal allergy. Salt water may not sound glamorous, but Dr. Sheldon Spector showed that certain patients obtain as much relief using salt water as with various drugs. The advantage of salt water is that it is physiologic. It's a natural liquid and can be used as often as you want for as long as you want.

Salt water may not work immediately, though, and you should allow a trial period of one or two weeks. Two common brands are Ocean Spray and Ayr-Mist.

2. Decongestants

Decongestants are designed to shrink your swollen mucous membranes and open your nasal passages. Depending on the brand you use, they can provide relief from four to twelve hours. Occasionally decongestants help with itching and sneezing, too.

However, decongestants are not a panacea. They can produce unwanted side effects such as stinging or burning. Some of them can actually increase your symptoms by causing a paradoxical swelling, called rebound. Although these sprays first shrink your nasal membranes, they then irritate them so much your membranes enlarge. Other side effects may be increasing your heart rate, raising your blood pressure, or making you jittery.

Don't let the warning about stinging, burning, elevated blood pressure, or rebound scare you. These effects occur only in a small percentage of the population. Furthermore, no long-term serious side effects from the use of decongestants have been reported. If a decongestant spray helps, you may use it. But, keep the following advice in mind. Although a lot of people tell me these rules are common sense, they are worth repeating.

- In order to determine whether decongestants elevate your blood pressure, ask your doctor to measure your blood pressure before and after you use these sprays.

- If you become jittery, nervous, experience an upset stomach, or if *anything* unusual happens while you are using a decongestant (or *any* medicine for that matter) stop the medicine and consult your doctor.

- If you don't obtain relief from your symptoms, stop the decongestant spray.

- If you obtain relief but subsequently a spray loses its effect, stop the spray.

- If a 12-hour spray lasts only one hour, stop the spray.

- If you have symptoms other than a stuffy nose (e.g. fever, vomiting, diarrhea, earache, sore throat, cough, wheezing, anything else), stop the spray and consult your doctor.

Common decongestants are:

Afrin
Coricidin Decongestant
Dristan
Duration
4-way
Neo-synephrine
NTZ
Otrivin
Privine
Sinex Decongestant

3. Cortisone Nasal Sprays

Recently, drug companies have introduced a number of cortisone nasal sprays. The companies claim the new brands of cortisone have fewer side effects and better effectiveness than the old types. In some cases they are correct. But, this is an individual matter. Each of you must try the sprays and decide for yourself.

Cortisone sprays can act instantly to relieve symptoms. This is an exception rather than the rule. Ordinarily, you must use cortisone nasal spray daily for up to three weeks just to start the effect. Then, you have to continue indefinitely to maintain the effect. Many people try a few squirts and give up because they do not get instant relief. With cortisone sprays, you must be patient.

I call cortisone nasal sprays "medicines for tomorrow" because you take them today to prevent tomorrow's problems. For *immediate* relief, you should use a decongestant.

Cortisone is an anti-inflammatory chemical. Thus, it is not specific for allergy. In fact, cortisone stops inflammation of *any* kind so it's also used for arthritis, burns, and certain cancers.

Be aware that cortisone nasal sprays can produce the identical dangerous side effects as cortisone pills. Cortisone is absorbed into your body when given in spray form. After a prolonged period of continual use, this can lead to the usual steroid side effects: weight gain, high blood pressure, psychological changes, cataracts, and ulcers. In children, cortisone can stunt growth. Some nasal sprays have a greater potential for causing such side effects than others. Your allergist can discuss this with you.

Some common cortisone nasal sprays are:

Beconase
Decadron Turbinaire
Nasacort
Nasalide
Vancenase

4. Cromolyn Nasal Spray (Nasalcrom)

In England in 1967, Dr. Roger Altounyan discovered the drug called cromolyn. This was heralded as a wonder drug because it prevented cells in the body from releasing the chemical mediators responsible for allergic symptoms. Doctors hoped that cromolyn would be the ultimate weapon in the fight against allergy, especially since cromolyn was not absorbed into the body and had no side effects.

As you might have guessed, it took awhile before cromolyn was approved for use in the United States. The name of the nasal spray is Nasalcrom. Like cortisone sprays, Nasalcrom is a "medicine for tomorrow." You need to use it two weeks to take effect. Then, you must use it *continually* to *prevent* your symptoms. Unfortunately cromolyn is not perfect and won't work in all of you.

Of further interest, cromolyn was approved for use in the eyes in early 1985. The eye drops are called Opticrom.

5. Atropine Nasal Spray

Ipratropium Bromide is an atropine-like chemical that you inhale every four or five hours. It's most helpful for preventing a runny nose. It doesn't help much with sneezing or stuffy nose.

6. Local Nasal Immunotherapy (LNIT)

Lastly, there is a nasal spray designed to treat the underlying cause of allergy. Researchers call this Local Nasal Immunotherapy. Doctors hoped it would replace traditional allergy injections. LNIT is not a drug or medicine. Rather, it is a technique to immunize your nose.

With traditional allergy injections, allergists give you an injection of grass, weed, or dust to force your body to make immunity. Eventually you make enough immunity so, upon exposure to allergens, you don't trigger your allergy symptoms.

Family doctors do the same thing when they immunize you or your children against polio and mumps. They inject the virus that they don't want you to get. But, they inject a *modified* form of the virus (called a vaccine), not the *really* infectious organism. This immunizes you. When the *real* polio or mumps virus comes around, your body is already protected because it has built its own immunity.

It was hoped that Local Nasal Immunotherapy would achieve the same results as allergy injections. By spraying increasing quantities of pollen into your nose, the theory was that the cells in your nose would make immunity and be protected from subsequent natural exposure.

So far, LNIT has not worked well. Doctors in New York and Michigan experimented with various doses using what they call "modified" pollen. The experiment was not a glorious success. Even if LNIT had worked, the researchers only tested for ragweed and grasses. If you had other allergies, you would be out of luck. Furthermore, the nasal drops were sometimes too strong and made people sneeze more.

The experiments are continuing, and you may read about them from time to time. But, there is a lot more work to be done.

Helpful hint 1: There are various categories of nasal spray. Within each category, there are many different brands.

Helpful hint 2: Nasal sprays have three purposes; to stop symptoms, prevent symptoms, or force your body to build immunity (Local Nasal Immunotherapy). Different ingredients are required to accomplish the different goals.

Helpful hint 3: Some nasal sprays are used on a one-time basis. Some sprays must be used continuously to achieve their effect.

Helpful hint 4: Many people think all nasal sprays are alike and don't know whether they are using cortisone, decongestants, saline, cromolyn, or atropine. Thus, they don't know what results to expect and therefore often misuse the sprays.

Unpleasant Side Effect Of Nasal Inhalers

We tend to think of nasal sprays as harmless. At one allergy conference Dr. Craig LaForce reported that two patients who had used a cortisone nasal spray for prolonged periods (one for fourteen months and the other for twenty-four months) perforated the cartilage material in the middle of their nose (called the nasal septum). A perforated septum means there is a hole in that middle part of your nose that separates your nose into right and left nostrils. Dr. LaForce's patients were using Vancenase (beclamethasone), but other doctors have reported similar perforations with Nasalide and Decadron.

Dr. LaForce thought that the combination of prolonged use and aiming the spray directly onto the nasal septum caused the perforation. But, he was not positive. Interestingly, one of the two patients was a nine year old child. The perforation was discovered when the child's parents reported hearing whistling sounds while the child slept. Air passing through the hole in the child's nose made the noise.

Helpful hint 1: Perforation of the nasal septum is a newly recognized possible side effect of the cortisone-type nasal inhalers.

Helpful hint 2: If you must use a nasal inhaler, don't aim it directly on your nasal septum.

Helpful hint 3: One drug company promoted a nasal cortisone spray by emphasizing that it alleviated allergies through a *direct* local action in the nose and not by a *systemic* effect exerted throughout the entire body. The company, which is a highly reputable one, wanted you to believe their nasal spray averted steroid side effects. While the beneficial effect probably *was* the result of local cortisone action, the claim is misleading. Nasal cortisone, like cortisone applied anywhere in the body, is *eventually* absorbed. Over a period of time this can cause the usual type of side effects from prolonged use. I suppose, though, that anything is fair in the game of advertising.

11

Asthma

According to the National Institutes of Health, over seventeen million people have asthma.

Many asthmatics are surprised to learn asthma can be due to allergy. The substances, such as pollens, dust, and animals, that irritate your nasal mucous membrane can irritate the membranes of your lungs, too. Foods can cause asthma reactions as well.

The following studies describe the latest findings. They add to our knowledge of what causes asthma and how to control it.

The topics covered are the current hot treatment for asthma, delayed asthma reactions, the risk of developing asthma when exposed to animals, how sinus infections can cause asthma, medications that can provoke asthma, a new inhalation technique to relieve asthma, a warning on over-diagnosis of asthma, negative ion generators, exercise and asthma, smoking and asthma, a new long lasting asthma inhaler, and when to use peak-flow meters.

Anti-inflammatory Drugs (Cortisones) Are the Hot Treatment for Asthma

Traditionally, doctors believed the primary reason you had asthma was due to tightening of the muscles that surround your bronchial tubes, thus narrowing these tubes so air cannot get in and out. To reverse this, they prescribed a medicine called a bronchodilator to relax those muscles and open the tubes, thus making your breathing easier.

In addition to tight bronchial muscles, irritation, mucus, and infection can obstruct your airways. When these other factors were significant, doctors prescribed cortisone since bronchodilators did not alleviate these other effects.

Now, doctors are reversing their stand and advocating treatment of inflammation and irritation first and constricted bronchial muscles second. This means cortisone is being recommended over bronchodilators. The recent national guideline on asthma treatment from the National Institutes of Health in Bethesda, Maryland, has strongly recommended this approach.

By now you know that cortisone has many serious and permanent side effects when used regularly. So, why the switch?

Since there are very few diseases where a particular treatment *always* works, doctors are constantly looking for an *ultimate* foolproof drug. To find such a drug, they, of course, study the people who don't respond to the standard treatment, which is euphemistically called the "treatment of choice."

When doctors study the non-responders, they invariably find a treatment that works. Thinking that if the new treatment worked in the resistant patients it ought to work in everyone, they then make broad and sweeping statements that they've found a new "treatment of choice."

Of course, eventually patients are found who don't respond to this new standard, either. This then sends the doctors in search of yet *another* standard.

In the case of steroids, doctors always knew steroids relieved asthma. But, since steroids are known to have serious side effects, they were reluctant to prescribe steroids until other, safer methods, like bronchodilators or getting rid of the cat, had been tried.

Now, as I said above, many physicians are advocating steroids from the beginning. If you want to know why, you'll have to ask them. I don't understand it.

Helpful hint 1: Although many physicians, including some from the prestigious National Institutes of Health, recommend steroids as the first drug to prescribe for asthma, steroids can have permanent and serious side effects. You should try safer methods first. However, if safer methods don't help, you have no choice but to take steroids.

Delayed Asthma Reactions

Most asthmatics react the moment they are exposed to an allergen. In some cases, though, there is a delay of up to twelve hours. This type of attack is called a Late Onset or Delayed Asthma Reaction. Doctors are beginning to realize that Late Onset Reactions occur more frequently than they had thought.

Sometimes Late Onset Reactions occur by themselves. Most often they occur several hours *after* an Immediate Onset Reaction.

Dr. R. Tamir from Israel proved that Late Onset Reactions can be triggered by exposure to plant pollens. Other doctors had previously shown they can be triggered by exposure to pets, chemicals, and foods.

Late Onset Reactions are not just a curiosity. When you develop asthma symptoms twelve hours after an exposure, it makes your diagnosis more difficult. If you and your doctors aren't aware of late reactions, you might disregard allergens you were exposed to earlier in the day. Unaware of these allergens, you would not make an effort to avoid them.

Treatment of Late Onset Reactions

The best treatment for Late Onset Reactions is avoidance of the offending substance. When that is not possible, you need to continue taking your medication long after an Immediate Reaction subsides to prevent a Late Onset Reaction from beginning. However, if you aren't aware of Late Onset Reactions, you might discontinue your medication too soon after an Immediate Onset Reaction ends and be caught unaware. Don't let this happen to you.

Helpful hint 1: Thanks to new research, doctors are aware of Late Onset Reactions. Understanding these reactions may help them treat many previously difficult cases of asthma.

Helpful hint 2: If you experience Late Onset Reactions, continue to take your medication from twelve to twenty-four hours after exposure even though you have no symptoms.

Helpful hint 3: Nasal and eye allergy symptoms can be delayed in their onset, too.

Risk Of Developing Asthma In Occupations Where There is Exposure To Animals

Many of you work with animals. And, many of you are rightly concerned that prolonged exposure to these animals might sensitize you and result in asthma. Although people who are constantly exposed to pets in their homes should be concerned too, they usually don't even want to think about this possibility.

Dr. Richard Evans studied how and when asthma began in 400 laboratory workers. He found certain individuals were at high risk. Those at greatest risk were allergic as children, had converted to a positive skin test to the animals they worked with, and showed a lung airway reaction when they breathed a drug called methacholine. The methacholine test is a method of detecting hyperreactive airways that are characteristic of asthma.

Dr. Evans' patients developed asthma from four months to two years after they began working with animals.

Helpful hint 1: Risk factors for developing asthma to animals include a history of allergy as a child, an asthmatic response to a test called methacholine challenge, and a positive skin test to the animal.

Helpful hint 2: After four years of exposure, only four of the 400 patients Dr. Evans studied developed asthma. So, the risk of asthma is not great. And, you should not be paranoid.

Sinus Infections Can Cause Asthma

If you have sinus disease and asthma, you will be more hopeful after you read about the research of Dr. Ray Slavin.

By vigorously treating sinus disease in certain asthmatics, Dr. Slavin found that his patients' asthma improved dramatically. Don't misunderstand this. He couldn't cure their asthma. But, he was able to lower the dose of medication they required to control their symptoms. Since many of his patients were on high doses of steroid-cortisone, this was a significant achievement.

Keep in mind that many patients who claim they have sinus disease do not actually have sinus disease. Furthermore, not all patients in Dr. Slavin's study who had sinus disease improved. Nevertheless the patients who did improve were so much better that this is worth looking into.

Even if clearing your sinuses doesn't help your asthma, at least your sinuses feel better.

Helpful hint 1: If you have asthma and sinus disease, ask your doctor to treat your sinus problem vigorously.

Asthma-Provoking Chemical Found In Medicine Used To Treat Asthma

This alarming discovery is a situation where the cure is worse than the disease. In this case, the cure actually *causes* the disease.

I don't know if you've read much about the sulfite controversy. Sulfite is a chemical preservative that's used to keep vegetables fresh, especially in salad bars. But sulfite is not restricted to salad bars. It's used as a general food preservative and even in some medications. Like many good things, though, sulfites can cause problems.

Severe asthmatics rely on mechanical respirators to inhale medication. When they pour these drugs into their respirator at the time of use, they are, obviously, exposing the drugs to air. So, manufacturers add a preservative to protect the drug's potency. This preservative is often the same bisulfite which is used on vegetables. Thus, susceptible asthmatics are aggravating their own symptoms.

The phenomenon is called Paradoxical Asthma because an asthmatic takes a drug to feel better, yet the preservative accompanying the drug makes them worse!

Don't panic. This applies only to bronchodilator solutions that are used in the motor-driven nebulizers. The common hand-held pressurized cannisters don't need this chemical, since the solutions in them are not exposed to air. Fortunately (and this is a lucky circumstance) only a few people react to the preservative. So, most of you can use these drugs without difficulty. However, if you use such medications and become worse after treatment, tell your doctor right away.

Hopefully, by the time you read this most drug companies will have removed the sulfites anyway.

Helpful hint 1: If you take any medication or treatment and notice your allergic symptoms become worse or that you experience side effects, stop the drug and consult your doctor.

Sudden Fatal Asthma With Open Airways

How can you have fatal asthma with *open* airways when, by definition, your airways are *closed* during an asthma attack?

To be honest, I don't know the answer.

Dr. Richard Nicklas reported on a group of asthmatics who were using asthma drugs called beta agonist bronchodilators. Although these drugs are effective in opening your airways, they can have a side effect of initiating an abnormal heart rhythm. This side effect can be severe enough to lead to cardiac arrest.

Interestingly, the fatalities Dr. Nicklas reported did *not occur* while these patients were in the *midst* of an asthma attack. Although these people had underlying asthma, at the time of their death their bronchial tubes were wide open *and* they were not having trouble breathing. Hence the fatality occurred "with open airways" since the death was actually due to cardiac arrest.

Despite the fact that the deaths occurred when there were no asthma symptoms, doctors named this condition Fatal Asthma. Since these deaths were due to heart disease and not asthma, I don't know why the doctors chose this name. To me, Fatal Irritable-heart Disease would be more appropriate.

So far, these deaths have only occurred in people who use excessive levels of beta agonists or in certain elderly people who cannot excrete these drugs quickly.

Helpful hint 1: Doctors sometimes attach strange names to diseases that tell you nothing about the disease or its underlying cause.

Helpful hint 2: Excessive levels of *any* drug, including vitamins and aspirin, can be dangerous.

Inhalation Technique For Asthmatics

Metered dose inhaler is the official name for the inhalers you puff when you have an attack of asthma. When you feel you have a band strapped across your chest so tightly you wonder how you'll get your next breath, you are supposed to squeeze the inhaler, take a deep breath so the medicine can fill your lungs, hold your breath for a few seconds, and then exhale. As you do this, you must aim the mouthpiece so the full dose of medication goes into your lungs instead of landing on the roof of your mouth or tongue where it would do no good.

If you think this is easy, think again. Picture someone at the end of a marathon where they are doubled over and gasping for breath. They must stop, pull out their inhaler, hold it steady while they direct it into their lungs, and inhale at the precise moment they squeeze the device. Then they must hold their breath for ten seconds as they allow the medicine to settle gently onto their airways.

Doctors realize inhaling correctly under the conditions of a severe attack is next to impossible, but until now no one had another idea. The new technique originated when someone put a tube, like the cardboard inside a roll of toilet paper, between the inhaling device and the mouth. When the inhaler is squeezed, the drug fills the tube which acts as a reservoir. Suddenly it was not so critical to aim the inhaler perfectly or inhale at precisely the right instant. With the drug in the tube, you could take your time and inhale several times to evacuate the contents of the tube.

After companies began supplying these tubes, called spacers, with their inhalers, researchers wondered whether the tubes helped. And, were they worth the extra cost?

Dr. John Toogood from Canada found the answer. He tested a group of patients and found half of them achieved better results with the extra tube. Half did not. His conclusion about how to tell which person would benefit and which would not? What do you think? Trial and error is the correct answer.

Helpful hint 1: For certain asthmatics a "spacer" placed between a metered dose inhaler and your mouth increases the effectiveness of delivering inhaled bronchodilator medicine to your lungs.

Helpful hint 2: If you are not obtaining satisfactory relief using an inhaler, try a spacer.

Helpful hint 3: Not every new development benefits every patient.

Spacers for Steroid/Cortisone Inhalers

Many asthmatics use metered dose *steroid* inhalers, which are similar in operation to bronchodilator inhalers, to deposit cortisone in their lungs. Doctors hoped that inhaling steroids *directly where they're needed* would achieve better results with fewer side effects than oral steroids which must traverse your entire body before they even reach your lungs. This would reduce the total dose of steroid delivered to you and hopefully cut down on long-term steroid side effects.

Although inhalers result in smaller amounts of steroids in your system, this technique deposits some of the drug in your mouth and on your vocal cords on its way to your lungs. This can result in an oral yeast infection called candidiasis. The symptoms are soreness of the mouth, irritation of the throat, and hoarseness.

Dr. Les Hendeles, who is a pharmacologist, reported that using a spacer, like the ones used when inhaling bronchodilators, prevents this from happening. He also found spacers can prevent the momentary cough some people experience when they inhale steroids.

Helpful hint 1: When doctors discover a new technique, like a spacer, they get excited and want to apply it to other situations. Sometimes the new idea actually works in the other situations.

Overdiagnosis And Overtreatment Of Black Asthmatics

In order to diagnose asthma, some doctors rely quite heavily on lung function tests. As you'd expect, they compare their patient's lung function to a normal standard. If their patient's test result is below normal, the doctors conclude that particular patient has asthma.

What would happen if the normal values were wrong? The answer: Doctors would make the wrong diagnosis.

This happened to several patients who were treated at Meharry Medical College. Two astute doctors realized that their clinic had been using a standard that was based on a group of White asthmatics. When the doctors investigated more thoroughly, they learned that Blacks had a different set of normal values. With this information, they reviewed their patients and identified those who had been diagnosed asthmatic but who were actually non-asthmatic.

The lung function test can also be used to decide how much asthma medicine an asthmatic should take. The more abnormal the test, the more medicine they'd require. Thus, if a Black person's dose was prescribed based on incorrect values, the person would be taking more medicine than necessary.

I don't want to leave the impression there has been widespread misdiagnosis and overtreatment. These cases involved only a few patients because doctors do not usually rely *solely* on lung function tests to make a diagnosis. Ordinarily, a thorough history, the right questions, and a good physical examination are all that's needed to diagnose asthma.

Helpful hint 1: If you are Black and were diagnosed asthmatic *solely* on the basis of a lung function test, ask your doctor to double check.

Negative Ion Generators For Treating Asthma

If you purchase an ion generator, don't expect it to help your asthma. A lot of people have already made this costly mistake. Their ion generators sit idly in their closets.

Although it may seem strange to you, changes in weather can trigger asthma. When this happens, people sometimes blame their symptoms on ions that are created in the air during periods of atmospheric turbulence.

As a result of this theory an industry sprang up manufacturing ion generators that would counteract the effect of the atmospherically-produced ions. Whether the theory was true or not, no one seemed to know or care. But, so many companies made this claim that Dr. Harold Nelson decided to study it.

Without disclosing what he was exposing them to, Dr. Nelson exposed asthmatic volunteers to negative and positive ions. The ions didn't affect his volunteers one way or the other. They weren't worse, and they weren't better.

Helpful hint 1: Asthma symptoms can flare when the weather changes. But, the increased symptoms patients experience are not due to ions in the air. There is another reason which doctors must still figure out.

Helpful hint 2: Ion generators won't make your asthma better or worse.

Discovery Of What Provokes Asthma After Exercise

Exercise triggers asthma in many patients. Because this is such a specific reaction, Drs. Regis McFadden and Sandra Anderson studied this condition hoping to learn how to treat all kinds of asthma more effectively. They've examined oxygen, carbon dioxide, sugar, and hormone levels. They reasoned that these substances change during exercise and therefore must be responsible for the symptoms.

As sometimes happens, this approach led nowhere. So, the doctors took a different approach and examined the effect of cooling and water loss from the lungs.

Dr. McFadden found *his* patients experienced bronchospasm due to cooling of the lungs. When you exercise, you breathe faster to dissipate your extra body heat. Dr. McFadden found asthma can begin when your lungs cool due to this evaporative water loss. The identical reaction occurs when cold air hits your lungs, again cooling your lungs.

Dr. Anderson found *her* patients, who live in Australia, experienced exercise-induced asthma due to loss of water from their lungs as they breathed faster, not because of associated heat loss.

Interestingly exercise-induced asthma can be prevented by using a device that warms the air as it enters your lungs or by altering the humidity of the inhaled air. Any of you who have exercise-induced wheezing may have noticed that running activities invariably trigger wheezing while swimming with your face in the water (high humidity) does not.

Helpful hint 1: Depending on the particular patient, exercise-induced wheezing is due to the rate of cooling or the rapid loss of water from the lungs.

Helpful hint 2: Exercise-induced wheezing is a specific entity and refers only to wheezing that occurs *after* exercise stops. Wheezing that begins *during* exercise is not generally considered to be the exercise kind.

Helpful hint 3: Sometimes scientists investigate a disease and uncover changes that have taken place such as the chemical changes that take place during vigorous exercise. But the changes may not turn out to be responsible for the disease. Instead these changes are labelled "associated findings" to emphasize that they do not indicate a cause-and-effect relationship.

Exercise-Induced Asthma Is Unrecognized

Dr. L. Kalish from Georgia examined exercise-induced asthma in high school athletes. Thirteen percent of the teenagers were found to have this condition. Although this seems like a high figure, other studies have shown comparable prevalence in other groups of people. For example, Dr. H. Dold of Illinois reported about 8 percent of the 1988 United States Olympic team were asthmatic.

As I mentioned previously, exercise-induced asthma produces wheezing, coughing, and tightness of the chest shortly *after* you exercise. If your symptoms occur *during* exercise, this is *not* exercise-induced asthma.

These findings are important because many children are undiagnosed and may be performing below their capability. However, when making this diagnosis, your doctors must be careful they aren't just dealing with lack of conditioning.

Helpful hint 1: Exercise-induced asthma has been found to occur in more children than previously thought.

Helpful hint 2: Exercise-induced asthma does not prevent outstanding achievement in sports. Many asthmatics become Olympic athletes despite this condition.

Asthma Worse If Family Member Smokes

Smoking can cause health problems for the person who smokes. It is now apparent that people who are merely exposed to cigarette smoke can suffer too.

Dr. Andrew Murray reported that children who have asthma have more symptoms when they're exposed to their parents' cigarette smoke. There was a noticeable effect in a closed, poorly ventilated room. This situation occurs especially in winter months (compared to the summer months) when your windows are likely to be closed and your children are likely to be playing indoors.

In previous studies doctors noted the same sort of effect occurred in offices where people work in a closed environment.

Helpful hint 1: No one has shown that smoking is beneficial to your health.

Helpful hint 2: For your own health and for the health of others, it's best to stop smoking.

Long-Lasting Inhaler For Asthma

At a company called Winthrop-Breon, researchers found a way to make metered dose asthma inhalers last longer than the usual four hours. The chemical they invented is bitolterol mesylate. The brand name is Tornalate.

Bitolterol mesylate is actually inactive. But, when you inhale it, one of your lung's enzymes breaks it into small molecules. One of these smaller molecules is a chemical called colterol. Colterol is an *active* drug from the same category as adrenaline, which is one of the most powerful anti-asthma drugs available.

The interaction between your lung's enzymes and the initially inactive drug makes bitolterol mesylate last up to eight hours. Unfortunately, in some of you, your lung's enzymes work twice as hard so bitolterol mesylate only lasts four hours, the same as the usual four-hour inhaled bronchodilator drugs.

Helpful hint 1: A clever scientist can alter a drug so that the drug helps you for a prolonged period of time.

Helpful hint 2: Sometimes the body is smarter than the smartest scientist and can ruin the best intentions.

Helpful hint 3: Some doctors prefer to prescribe aerosol bronchodilators. Others prefer tablet or liquid preparations.

Helpful hint 4: If you use an inhaled bronchodilator, you may want to try the long-acting kind. They might reduce the frequency with which you must use your inhaler and make it easier to control your asthma.

Peak-Flow Meters

Allergists usually encourage you to match the amount of medication you take with the severity of your symptoms. So, the more severe your asthma, the more medicine you use. The less severe your asthma, the less medicine you use.

To gauge how much you need, your doctor may ask you to assess your asthma symptoms by measuring the amount of air you can exhale into a measuring device called a peak-flow meter. When doing this, you keep a daily diary. By comparing your results to a standard value, you learn how your lungs are functioning so you can take the appropriate amount of medication. If your peak-flow declines, you take more drugs. If your peak-flow approaches normal, you take less drugs.

The main advantage is that a peak-flow meter can give you an early warning of impending severe asthma. Thus forewarned, you can theoretically prevent runaway asthma, which could lead to status asthmaticus and the need for hospitalization.

Despite the hoopla about peak-flow meters, there is another way to tell how much medicine you need. If you cough, wheeze, feel tightness of the chest, wheeze during exercise, or wake up at night coughing, you need more medicine. In most individuals these symptoms are as good a test of lung function as peak-flow meters. However, when using your symptoms to guide you, you *have to pay attention to your body*. Some of you may not want to be bothered thinking about what's happening to you. In that case, you should think about getting a peak-flow meter.

Helpful hint 1: If you need a number to tell you whether you are coughing, wheezing, having tightness of the chest, or waking up at night with asthma, buy and use a peak-flow meter.

12

Allergy and Pregnancy

Pregnancy is a time when a woman's body undergoes changes. Thus, it should come as no surprise that during pregnancy allergies can begin, stay the same, become worse, or even improve. There is no test to predict which way allergy will go in your case. The first study discusses this issue.

The next two studies explain that a pregnant woman who receives allergy injections does not harm the fetus and may even be immunizing her unborn child.

Asthma Symptoms During Pregnancy

Allergists and obstetricians know that pregnancy can aggravate nasal allergies and asthma. This does not happen to all women or even most women, but it is not uncommon either.

Dr. Michael Schatz surveyed over 300 women and found the outlook is not as bad as you might have imagined. Most women did not even develop asthma during pregnancy. Of those who already had asthma and became worse, 75 percent reverted to their original level after they delivered their child. This showed that the exacerbation of asthma during pregnancy was only a temporary situation.

Furthermore, Dr. Schatz found that women who become worse do not become progressively more severe with each pregnancy. They simply become worse, revert to baseline, get worse, revert to baseline, and so forth.

Helpful hint 1: There is no need to panic if your asthma becomes worse when you are pregnant. There's a good chance your symptoms will subside after you deliver.

Helpful hint 2: However, you have no justification for complacency if your asthma improves while you are pregnant. Your symptoms may return. This happened to several women in Dr. Schatz's study.

Allergy Injections Do Not Sensitize The Fetus

Previous studies have shown that allergy injections do not increase the incidence of congenital abnormalities or difficult labor. This is to be expected since allergy injections don't contain drugs or chemicals, just extracts of grasses, trees, weeds, pets, and dust. These are substances that enter your body whether or not you receive injections.

Since doctors are born worriers, though, they wondered whether injections might harm the fetus, even though allergy injections had already been shown not to harm the mother.

Dr. David Graft studied a group of mothers who were receiving injections of honey bee venom. The mothers had been found sensitive to bees and were receiving injections to immunize them against bee stings.

After the mothers delivered, the doctors tested the infants and found the children had not been sensitized to bee venom.

Thus, allergy injections during pregnancy are safe for *both* mother and fetus.

Helpful hint 1: Since allergy injections contain only natural substances (i.e. no drugs or medications) one would not think allergy injections would be harmful to the fetus or detrimental to pregnancy. Scientific studies confirm this.

Fetus Protected Against Allergy When Mother Gets Shots

In another study, the previously mentioned Dr. Michael Schatz was one of a group of doctors at the Kaiser Hospital in San Diego who studied newborns whose mothers had received allergy injections during pregnancy. He and his co-workers discovered that the mothers had transferred some of their immunity to the fetus. Although doctors already knew injections weren't harmful, this was the first report showing injections were helpful to a fetus.

Before taking this study as gospel truth, you should wait for confirming evidence from other investigators. Nevertheless this is encouraging news.

Helpful hint 1: A mother's immunizing injections seem to bolster the immunity of the fetus.

13

Penicillin Allergy

Drug reactions are increasingly common in modern medicine. Statistics show nearly one out of ten hospitalized patients experience a reaction to one of the drugs they are given.

Possibly the most common allergic-type drug reaction is to penicillin. However, penicillin has important benefits, so scientists have devoted a great deal of time to studying penicillin allergy. This research has enabled doctors to understand how drug reactions occur and how to treat such reactions.

You will read three studies about penicillin allergy. The first study describes how penicillin allergy can be circumvented. The second describes a new test for penicillin allergy. The third one is disappointing, though. It shows that massive screening of the general population for penicillin allergy would be futile.

Penicillin Allergy No Longer A Widespread Threat

So many of you have been told you're allergic to penicillin that researchers have devoted an enormous amount of time and money searching for a way to enable you to use penicillin anyway.

There are five answers to the problem. Two of the answers are new, and three are old.

1. One of the answers comes from Dr. Dorothy Sogn's studies. She reported that most of you who believe you are allergic to penicillin are not *really* allergic to it. She took histories, did examinations, and tested patients who claimed they were sensitive. She discovered that 75 percent of you have been misdiagnosed. Thus, many of you are not allergic to penicillin and have no reason to avoid it.

2. The second answer is a simple bit of wisdom. If you're allergic to penicillin, use *another* antibiotic. Fortunately there are many antibiotics which kill bacteria effectively, so you aren't wedded to penicillin. Of course, a corollary of this rule is: Don't use *any* antibiotic unless you *truly* need it. The more often you use an antibiotic the greater the chance you may wind up becoming allergic to it.

3. The third answer is: If you absolutely need penicillin, but are allergic to it, your doctor can treat you beforehand with anti-allergy medicines. This would prevent a reaction from getting out of control or even prevent a reaction in the first place.

4. The fourth technique has been known for years. If you have a particular infection where nothing but penicillin will do, such as certain infections of the heart or bones,

you can be hospitalized. There, you can be given penicillin intravenously in gradually increasing doses until you reach the amount that kills bacteria (the therapeutic level). This desensitizes you so you don't react.

5. Finally, the fifth method was described by Dr. Barbara Stark from Texas. She gave penicillin by mouth, according to a specific schedule, and showed how allergic patients could be desensitized orally instead of intravenously. Since you need a strict schedule and careful monitoring to do this successfully, don't try it on your own.

Helpful hint 1: The majority of you who think you are allergic to penicillin are not.

Helpful hint 2: If you are truly allergic to penicillin, you can usually take the drug after a simple desensitization course.

Helpful hint 3: Don't take antibiotics (or any other drug) unnecessarily.

Helpful hint 4: If you are desensitized to penicillin, this is not a lifetime cure. Desensitization would have to be repeated every time you wished to use penicillin.

Tests for Penicillin Allergy

Dr. Louis Mendelson from Connecticut solved a knotty problem in penicillin allergy. When allergists test for penicillin allergy, they must use two different chemicals.

One of them, called Minor Determinant Mixture, is unstable.

Strictly speaking, Minor Determinant Mixture is supposed to be made fresh according to a particular process, but some doctors make their own by placing penicillin in an alkaline solution at room temperature. The penicillin breaks down under these conditions. This material is not identical to Minor Determinant Mixture, but it is similar. When used for testing, this material is about 65 percent accurate. The scientifically-made mixture is 95 percent accurate.

Dr. Mendelson and his co-worker developed a freeze-dried Minor Determinant Mixture. Freeze-drying protects the potency and allows the scientifically-made material to be shipped anywhere. A doctor who used this freeze-dried Minor Determinant Mixture would be able to tell you your *exact* chance of having penicillin allergy.

Helpful hint 1: If you have been tested for penicillin allergy, ask if both Major and Minor Determinant Mixtures were used.

Helpful hint 2: If Minor Determinant Mixture was used, ask whether your doctors made it themselves. If the mixture was made by your doctors, the results are only 65 percent accurate.

Helpful hint 3: A drug company is trying to manufacture freeze-dried Minor Determinant Mixture so it will be available to all doctors throughout the United States.

Testing For Penicillin Allergy Has Limited Value

While studying penicillin allergy, Dr. Timothy Sullivan showed that *routine* massive testing for penicillin allergy can be a waste of time.

With the availability of both Major and Minor Determinant Mixtures, physicians who have access to these testing materials can diagnose penicillin allergy with great accuracy. However, even if tests show you aren't allergic, this does not mean you won't *become* allergic at some time in the future. The more penicillin you use, the greater the chance you can become allergic. You would have to be re-tested each time you wanted to use penicillin to make sure you had not converted between the time you were previously tested and the present time.

Helpful hint 1: Testing for penicillin allergy is accurate when the correct test materials are used.

Helpful hint 2: Testing you for penicillin allergy determines your state of sensitivity *at the moment in time the test is performed*. These tests are not crystal balls and do not predict or guarantee your *future* state of sensitivity.

Helpful hint 3: When Minor Determinant Mixture becomes available, there will be extensive testing for penicillin allergy. Then, many people will falsely believe they are protected from being allergic to penicillin for the rest of their life, despite the fact that the test only discloses their *current* degree of sensitivity.

Helpful hint 4: Wishful thinking sometimes over-whelms common sense.

14

Bee Sting Allergy

Due to the pain, swelling, and soreness of a bee sting, you are wise to keep a safe distance from bees even if you aren't allergic. When allergy is involved, avoiding bee stings is a necessity. A sting to an allergic individual can mean the difference between life and death.

When bees sting you, they inject about ten different chemicals into your body. Certain of these chemicals are toxic and cause pain, redness, swelling, and itching *at the site* of the sting. If the stinger is dirty, you can also develop an infection *at the site* of the sting.

However, if you are allergic, you develop symptoms *far away* from the sting; hives, asthma, and, in extreme cases, fatal shock.

Those of you who are truly allergic must often undertake a long series of immunizing injections to protect yourself against the fatal kind of allergic bee sting reactions.

The first study explains that immunizing injections for bee stings, like the injections for pollens, dust, animals, and molds, do not necessarily continue indefinitely. The second study unmasks the myth about killer bees which are terrorizing certain parts of the United States.

Bee Sting Injections Need Not Last Forever

In 1979 there was a mini-revolution in treating bee sting allergy. For years Dr. Mary Loveless had pleaded with allergists to inject bee venom instead of whole-body extract when treating bee sting allergy. Most of the medical community ignored her because whole-body extract seemed to be as effective as the venom. Furthermore whole-body extract had the advantage of being easier to make and inexpensive to give.

After spending hundreds of hours reviewing the old studies and after several years of performing new studies, doctors at Johns Hopkins Hospital discovered that Dr. Loveless had been right. Venom was superior. Therefore, despite the higher cost, allergists switched their patients to venom.

Treatments begin with approximately twenty injections to build the dose to a protective level of immunity. This is generally followed by monthly injections to maintain your immunity. Since no one knew with certainty how long the immunity would last, until now the injections have been recommended indefinitely.

Recently Drs. Robert Reisman and Martin Valentine discovered that you do not have to continue bee venom shots forever. Certain children and adults are permanently immunized after only three years of treatment. Children were more successful stopping shots after three years than adults.

Before you stop injections on your own, though, consult your doctor. Allergists can help you figure out whether you are one of the lucky ones that can stop after three years.

Remember, too, that people who experience *local* reactions don't need treatment at all. The definition of bee sting allergy is a *systemic* reaction. In other words, you react someplace other than where you are stung. When you swell up horribly or have a lot of pain at the site of the sting, this is not allergy in the medical sense. To be allergic, you must break out in hives, have asthma, have trouble swallowing, or collapse. Local itching, swelling, and pain don't count.

After taking your medical history, if your allergists are still not sure whether you're allergic, they can figure it out by doing skin tests for bee venom.

Helpful hint 1: You have the best chance for achieving a permanent cure for bee sting allergy if you take injection treatment as a child.

Helpful hint 2: Each case treated with bee venom injections must be examined *individually* to decide when injections may be stopped.

Helpful hint 3: Bee sting allergy refers to generalized or systemic reactions, not to local reactions or infections which occur at the site of the sting.

Killer Bee Threat Is Overdramatized

Newspaper editors love a good scary item. The story of the killer bees that have invaded the United States is made for their headlines.

Killer bees are bees that originally came from outside the United States. They are bigger and more aggressive than domestic bees. When angry, they sting in swarms instead of one at a time.

But do they kill? And do they cause allergic reactions? These bees don't really kill people. They fly in groups. And, when they are angry several of them sting you at the same time.

When it comes to allergy, they are not more dangerous than domestic bees. In fact they are less dangerous. Dr. J. E.

Lowry found killer bee venom sacs are smaller and therefore contain less venom than domestic bees. So, there is less chance of a fatal allergic reaction from a single killer bee than a single domestic bee sting.

Helpful hint 1: In allergy, the larger the dose of allergens you receive, the worse your reaction will be. Since killer bees have less venom than domestic bees, you have less chance of a severe *allergic* reaction from killer bees than from domestic bees.

Helpful hint 2: Stay away from killer bees. They are mean and ornery.

15

New Diseases

Although you might think physicians know everything because they can clone genes, alter viruses, and transplant vital organs, they are still discovering new ailments. The following reports are about diseases which have recently been shown to be caused by allergy.

The first two studies describe allergic reactions that occur after exercise. The third study describes how an artificial sweetener can cause hives. The fourth is a new definition of chronic hives. This is followed by a study that tells you about occupational diseases that are due to allergy. The final two reports describe conditions that mimic allergy to illustrate the point that not every sneeze is allergy.

Hives And Swelling During Exercise

Have you ever exercised and broken out in hives or gotten itchy? I know this sounds weird, but it happens to some people. Although these kinds of reactions have probably occurred for years, soon after Dr. Albert Sheffer wrote about them in a medical journal, there was a rash (excuse the expression) of such cases.

Exercise reactions are a fascinating problem, especially when you consider how much we exercise to stay healthy. People with this condition get hives, itching, asthma, and even collapse when their bodies become warm during vigorous athletics. What is truly unbelievable is that some of these patients only experience these reactions if they eat a specific food (it's a different food for different people) *before* they exercise. Even more strange is that some only suffer if they eat that particular food *after* they exercise. Would you believe that celery, which seems so innocuous to me, was the offending food in several cases?

Treatments are available, but just the idea of such an illness is remarkable.

Helpful hint 1: If you experience unusual symptoms during or shortly after exercise, see your family doctor or allergist.

Exercise Can Be Harmful

Soon after Dr. Albert Sheffer reported about the skin and asthma reactions that occur after exercise, Dr. R. Sabinsky interviewed long distance runners in a New York race and found almost 50 percent of them experienced nasal symptoms after exercise.

Helpful hint 1: Although regular exercise is healthy, in certain individuals exercise produces allergic-type reactions.

Helpful hint 2: Exercise can provoke hives, nasal allergy, and asthma in susceptible individuals.

Trigger Of Chronic Hives

Chronic hives and itching are extremely annoying. Many times the culprit cannot be found. So, when scientists discover a new cause, it is of great interest.

Dr. A. Kulczycki at Washington University Medical School reported several cases of hives and itching which he traced to the artificial sweetener aspartame (Nutrasweet). This type of reaction is very uncommon. But, if you have hives or itching, consider stopping aspartame on a trial basis.

Helpful hint 1: Certain chemicals which are innocuous to the majority of the population can cause allergic reactions in selected individuals.

Helpful hint 2: Although aspartame may provoke an allergic reaction in select individuals, there is no need to ban this substance entirely. The majority of the population tolerates it with no ill effect.

Definition of Chronic Hives

Dr. Alan Kaplan has studied hives for most of his medical career. So, he's considered a world-class authority, a kind of guru of hives. Previously, hives were defined as chronic when they persisted more than six weeks. Acute meant they lasted less than six weeks even though six weeks is a long time when you can't sleep at night due to itching and are scratching your skin raw during the day.

Now, Dr. Kaplan has determined that the six-week definition is misleading. Since proper treatment depends so much on correct diagnosis, allergists must change their thinking.

According to Dr. Kaplan, acute hives should refer to hives which last one or two hours, go away, and then perhaps come back in a different location on your body. Thus, it is *not how many weeks* you have hives that matters. It is how long each hive persists at its location on your body. So, even if you've suffered with hives for months, if your hives move around a lot, this indicates the acute type for diagnostic, and therefore therapeutic, purposes.

When hives remain in the *same* location for hours at a time, this is chronic hives, even if you've only been symptomatic a few weeks.

This may seem like semantics to you, but the reason hives behave differently is due to the underlying cause. And, knowing the underlying cause leads to more appropriate and effective treatment.

Helpful hint 1: Sometimes just changing the definition of an illness can help your doctors understand a disease process. And, better understanding leads to more effective treatment.

Occupational Allergies

The United States has a heavily industrialized economy. As a result, thousands of you are exposed to a bewildering array of chemicals. As companies seek to discover new and better products to compete in the world marketplace, they create even more chemicals. Every chemical created is a potential allergen to someone. If the right person and the right allergen come together, allergy symptoms are inevitable.

People who have occupational allergies can experience such symptoms as rashes, itching, sneezing, wheezing, coughing, headaches, and fatigue. Some of you may only be ill at work. But, some symptoms persist and can even begin hours after you leave the workplace. So, even if your symptoms are worse at home, they could still have originated from exposure at work.

Occupational allergy is a fascinating subject. Each industry has its own quirks. To describe all these problems in a small book would be impossible. Nevertheless you might be interested in a short list of chemicals that have been implicated in occupational allergy.

platinum salts
nickel salts
trimellitic anhydride
mealworm
himic anhydride
phthalic anhydride
ethylene oxide
bee pollen

freon
sunflower pollen
toluene diisocyanate
hexamethonium isocyanate
poultry farm material
moth scale
peach skin

When health and safety engineers sound a warning about occupational exposure and its dangers, think what they are saying. There is a difference between a *toxic irritant* and an *allergic* effect. With toxicity, symptoms are due to *high levels* of chemicals. These levels are unsafe to everyone, whether you are allergic or nonallergic. For example, high levels of chlorine or acid in a swimming pool will burn, irritate, and even cause blindness. The *normal* level of chlorine and acid in a pool is safe and actually protects you against illnesses caused by infectious organisms.

Allergy, on the other hand, occurs when substances are present at virtually *undetectable* levels. Therefore, although the levels would be considered safe according to toxic guidelines, the allergic person is still suffering. This is because the allergic person has excess IgE antibody which makes the "safe" level a problem.

Helpful hint 1: There are a multitude of chemicals you are exposed to at home and on the job. These chemicals can cause toxic reactions in *anyone* when present at high levels. When present at virtually undetectable levels, these chemicals can cause allergic symptoms in certain *susceptible individuals*.

Helpful hint 2: Most of the time (and this is important to keep in mind) chemicals do not cause symptoms at the levels at which most of you are exposed.

Helpful hint 3: If you have symptoms at work, consult your doctors. They can help you decide whether or not your symptoms are work-related.

Gustatory Rhinitis

Have you ever wondered why your nose runs when you eat spicy foods?.

Dr. Michael Kaliner was curious whether this was related to allergy. Upon studying this process, Dr. Kaliner found that spicy foods contain capsaicin. This chemical is responsible for producing a runny nose.

Interestingly, Dr. Kaliner uses capsaicin to study nasal physiology. He needed a reliable method to stimulate mucus so he could analyze how the nose functions. If you volunteer to be a subject in his laboratory, you can eat all the spicy food you want and get paid for doing it.

Helpful hint 1: Not all runny noses are due to allergy.

Non-allergic Eosinophilic Rhinitis

Eosinophils are cells in the body which are known to be the hallmark of allergy. So, when Dr. Michael Mullarkey found a group of patients who had eosinophils in their nasal membrane, but had negative allergy tests, no history of allergy, and no response to anti-allergy medication, this was big news in allergy circles. This may not seem important to you, but it is to allergists.

Since many of these subjects were being treated for allergy, Dr. Mullarkey concluded that many people who are diagnosed with nasal allergy (rhinitis) may not really be allergic. As you know, allergy tends to get blamed for many events, even when it is not at fault. For example, children often say they are allergic to spinach just so they don't have to eat it.

Other reasons for non-allergic nasal symptoms are the common cold, overuse of nasal sprays, irritants in the air, changes in climate, certain nasal polyps, various drugs, pregnancy, and hypothyroidism.

Dr. Mullarkey's report is important because it reminds all of us, doctors and patients alike, that a *correct* diagnosis is the best hope for effective treatment.

Helpful hint 1: Not all sneezes are due to allergy.

16

House Dust Control and The Home Environment

Allergy to house dust is common. Contrary to what you may think, the dust that causes allergic problems is not simply dirt that you find on the ground. Allergic-type house dust is made of plant by-products such as cotton, kapok, mold particles, and insects such as house dust mite and cockroaches.

If you have an indoor pet, you might think to include animal dander and saliva in the amorphous mixture that forms allergic-type house dust. But strictly speaking, pets are a different category, which is why I put them in their own chapter earlier in this book.

The following studies illuminate little-known facts about the best methods to control allergy to house dust mites, the effectiveness of air purifiers, and problems that have been reported due to home insulation.

House Dust Mite Allergy

House dust mites are microscopic insects that live in rugs and in the cotton and kapok stuffing material used in mattresses, boxsprings, pillows, and chairs. Allergists love to show you a greatly magnified picture of a dust mite (Dermatophagoides Pteronyssimus) because the insects look so scary. They produce material which can enter the air you breathe and provoke allergy if you're susceptible. Below are observations of Drs. Thomas Platts-Mills and Richard Lockey about how to control allergy to mites and prevent allergic reactions to these insects.

Dr. Platts-Mills reported that he was able to rid a house of dust mites using a chemical called primiphos methyl. A single treatment lasted up to six weeks. Benzyl benzoate and tannic acid have also helped to varying degrees. Dr. Richard Lockey showed that caffeine is another chemical that can effectively lower the concentration of mites in your home.

Another well-known way to reduce the mite population is to maintain the humidity below 50 percent. Mites don't breed well in low humidity. The fewer the mites, the fewer the symptoms they can trigger in you.

Finally, many doctors even recommend a program of immunizing injections to build your resistance to mites.

Helpful hint 1: House dust mites can provoke allergic symptoms in susceptible individuals.

Helpful hint 2: No matter how strong your skin test reaction to dust mites, you will not experience symptoms unless mites are in your environment. So, in parts of the United States where the lack of humidity prevents mites from growing, mites can't affect you.

Helpful hint 3: As is true with most allergenic substances, there are various ways of coping. With dust mite allergy, you can lower the humidity, use chemicals to kill them, or get allergy-immunizing injections.

Helpful hint 4: If you use a chemical to kill insects such as dust mites, be careful that you don't react to the chemical itself.

Helpful hint 5: If you are allergic to house dust mite but mite allergy is a small part of your total problem, you're better off spending your time and energy taking care of the other allergens first.

Helpful hint 6: If you don't want to use chemicals with strange names to kill mites, you can spill coffee, which contains caffeine, on your rug (only joking!).

Effectiveness Of Air Cleaners

There are two types of air cleaning machine. Each contains a fan which blows air through a special cleansing unit. One machine cleans by blowing air through a sponge-like material called High Efficiency Particle Absorbent (HEPA). The other machine contains two electrified metal plates. As room air passes through the machine, the plates attract and hold small particles. This is called electrostatic cleaning.

According to engineers, both types of machine are effective at cleaning air. But, allergists are only interested in how much better you feel and not necessarily how clean the air is. You'd think cleaning air and helping you would be the same. It turns out they are not.

Upon investigation of homes with air cleaners, Dr. Charles Reed found shelves were cleaner, floors looked better, and patients had to do less dusting. But, only one-fourth of the patients improved. Needless to say, this was very disappointing to Dr. Reed.

This finding is surprising until you think about it. The reasons for the lack of improvement are:
- filters clog when air cleaners are run continuously,
- you are usually allergic to outdoor substances, too,
- and, you can't isolate yourself in your house all day since you can't conduct your life in a bubble.

Helpful hint 1: Air cleaners might do a wonderful job cleaning your house, but they aren't necessarily effective in relieving your allergy symptoms.

Helpful hint 2: Since air cleaners are not guaranteed to help allergy, you should use them on a trial basis to see if they're worth purchasing.

Helpful hint 3: People ought to know better than to expect much help from a treatment that is directed at one facet of a multifaceted problem.

Facts On Exposure To Home Insulation

Some people believe that home insulating material which is made from urea-formaldehyde can produce harmful vapors that trigger allergic symptoms. Until recently, though, no one had surveyed the population to learn the prevalence of this kind of problem.

Out of curiosity, several doctors in Canada tested the adverse effects of urea-formaldehyde in a controlled environment. They studied a group of patients who swore vehemently that urea-formaldehyde vapors from home insulation triggered their asthma. By placing these subjects in a special chamber, the doctors were able to examine them before and after exposure to vapor from this kind of insulation.

The surprising result was that only one of the subjects got worse. The rest did not develop asthma despite their previous assertions that formaldehyde bothered them. The experiment showed that urea-formaldehyde is not as big a problem as was originally believed.

The research also illustrated the fact that doctors must always double-check their patients' observations and suspicions when it comes to determining which substances are responsible for allergic reactions. If a patient's suspicion isn't correct, a doctor is obliged to look for the real culprit. Assuming a suspicion is correct, no matter how strongly a patient believes in it, would lull both physician and patient into a false sense of security that they've made the correct diagnosis and are doing everything possible to achieve relief.

Helpful hint 1: Home insulating material is not the culprit it was thought to be.

17

Miscellaneous

The following studies discuss several topics in allergy. They answer frequently-asked questions about sinus headaches, a new approach to the treatment of itchy, watery eyes, a new theory about how to avoid allergens, why allergy symptoms are often worse at night, a surprising fatality due to ingestion of honey bee pollen, the worst location for allergy in the United States, some comments on how to tell which is the worst year for allergies, the problem of allergy to X-ray contrast material, a study on allergy to latex gloves, and finally a curious case where a woman was truly allergic to her husband.

Look at the list of topics in the table of contents to find the subjects that interest you. For your general information, though, you should read everything. You will learn principles you can apply to many questions that arise in allergy.

Hope For Sinus Headache Sufferers

There are uncountable people who have headaches due to sinus disease. Dr. Sheldon Spector selected a typical group of such patients and investigated them thoroughly.

Your sinuses are located deep inside your skull bone. The only way your doctors can tell what is happening in them is either open your skull, which is a major surgical operation, or order an X-ray.

Dr. Spector hoped he could find an easy, inexpensive method such as a carefully taken history, a physical examination, looking at your sinuses with a flashlight in a dark room, which is a technique used to visualize fluid in the sinuses, ordering blood tests, or obtaining nasal and sinus bacterial cultures. He even tried special fiberoptic instruments. Lastly, he and his co-workers tried to feel the sinuses by pressing over the forehead and cheeks.

After all this work, Dr. Spector discovered that *none* of these methods was guaranteed. Since an operation to open your skull would be overkill, an X-ray turned out to be the only *accurate* way to make the diagnosis.

At first, this might strike you as discouraging news. On the contrary, the news is encouraging. Even if your head hurts, unless you have had an X-ray proving your sinuses are abnormal, you may not have sinus disease. And, if you don't have sinus disease, you should stop being treated for sinus disease. Instead, you should find out what is *really* causing your headaches. You achieve nothing by treating a sinus problem that isn't there. Such treatment merely distracts you from diagnosing and treating the *true* cause of your headache.

Helpful hint 1: If you don't *truly* have sinus disease, there's no point being treated for sinus disease. Instead, find out what you have and treat *that*.

Helpful hint 2 By the time you finish this book, I hope you've learned that you should not be treated for one disease when your problem is caused by another disease.

Treatment Found For Itchy, Watery Eyes

One of the symptoms of hay fever is itchy, watery eyes. Two doctors from the Netherlands discovered a new way to stop these symptoms. The doctors noticed that 75 percent of their patients who had eye symptoms improved upon using medication that is usually prescribed for nasal symptoms.

Dr. Pelikan, one of the doctors who performed the study, believes that when the nasal membrane is strongly affected by allergy, the inflammation caused by the allergic reaction travels backward from the nose to the eyes through the tear ducts. Ordinarily these ducts carry your tears the other way, from your eyes down into your nose. Thus, by treating nasal allergy, Dr. Pelikan alleviated eye symptoms.

Helpful hint 1: Some patients who have allergic conjunctivitis (the official name for eye allergy) are symptomatic due to retrograde nasal allergy.

Helpful hint 2: If you have persistent allergy symptoms despite treatment, return to your doctors so they can figure out why you aren't responding.

How To Avoid Allergens

Do you know what priming is? This is a concept that was promulgated years ago. You should become familiar with it. Understanding priming will help you understand a new philosophy of avoiding allergens.

When you are allergic to more than two substances, exposure to one of them may prime you to be more sensitive to the other.

For example, if one morning you walk among trees and return home to play with your cat, you'll be more ill than if you just play with your cat. You could say that once tree pollen started your ball rolling, the slightest cat exposure triggered an allergy avalanche.

Another way of looking at priming is to think of allergy as the straw that broke the camel's back. If you pile straw on a camel's back, as the aphorism says, the camel will bear the load until the breaking point. When the last straw is placed, the one that is too much for the camel, the poor camel's back will break. At first you may think that the *last* straw was the one responsible for breaking the camel's back, but *all* the straws contributed equally.

It is important to understand priming in order to understand a new concept in avoiding allergens.

Since it takes a combination and accumulation of allergens (priming) to make you ill, it's possible for you to obtain relief by removing only a few of the many allergens to which you are allergic. Since all the straws contribute equally to breaking the camel's back, you could lighten the camel's load by removing *any* of the straws. Of course the more straws you remove the lighter the load, but technically it isn't necessary to remove every last wisp unless you have an extraordinarily weak camel.

This is a long-winded way of stating that you don't need to undertake every known form of treatment in order to obtain relief. More important, each of you can choose which form of treatment (which straw) you want to remove.

Dr. John Conell studied priming and showed that many allergy sufferers could eliminate two or three substances and improve enough to ignore the other allergens to which they reacted. This did not mean they achieved 100 percent relief. On average, his patients achieved about 80 percent relief. But, this was more than satisfactory since they were then able to lead a normal life without going overboard on allergy treatment.

The Old Way To Think Of Allergy Treatment

In the old days allergists wrote a prescription for your life, not just for your medication.

- If you're allergic to trees, move to the beach.
- If you're allergic to ragweed, go to Europe.
- If you're allergic to cats, get rid of your cats.
- If you're allergic to grass, stay indoors.
- If you have asthma, quit sports.
- If you're allergic to dust, scrub the house daily.

Although this sort of advice is technically correct, it may not be the optimal solution for you. There are so many variables of lifestyle, habits, and personality traits that a knee-jerk answer is not appropriate. That is why a computer will never be able to replace a good old-fashioned doctor who has your *overall* best interest at heart.

The New Way To Think Of Allergy Treatment

The concept of priming shows you a sensible way to overcome your allergy. Previously you might have thought you had no choices. After seeing an allergist, you would be told your sensitivities and be expected to avoid the offending allergens or automatically start a series of allergy injections.

In the new method, you consider your entire picture; your allergens, symptoms, lifestyle, and preferences. Then decide which of your various allergens to treat. If you can do a good job on a few of them, you may improve so much that you can ignore other allergens which are more difficult to deal with. You'd be surprised how often you can lead a normal life with just a few minimal adjustments.

Helpful hint 1: You can often do a few simple things for a limited number of allergens and feel so much better that undertaking additional treatment is not worth the extra effort.

Helpful hint 2: In allergy, you can choose which of the various treatment possibilities you wish to undertake.

Helpful hint 3: The medically and scientifically best treatment may not be the *personally* best treatment for *you.*

Why Allergy Symptoms Are Often Worse At Night

Many allergy patients feel worse at night. Dr. Michael Smolensky at the University of Texas tried to find out the reason, but he could not discover a *single* factor that explained all cases.

In some patients Dr. Smolensky found that increased symptoms were due to a person's more intense exposure to household allergens, such as dust, pets, and feathers, which they are exposed to in the evening when they are at home.

In others he found the protective level of adrenal hormone had dropped during the night and allowed allergy symptoms to surface. Adrenal hormones normally decrease at night, but in allergy patients this decrease can precipitate an adverse effect. The effect is so well known that some people have mistakenly concluded that adrenal hormone deficiency causes allergy in the first place. Although intriguing, this idea has been proven completely false.

Another contributing factor was an increase in reactivity of the lung's airways that occurs in some patients at night.

Thus, those of you who are worse at night must consult your doctors and investigate your *particular* reason for nighttime symptoms. Only by doing this can you learn how to control your allergies effectively.

Helpful hint 1: If your allergies are worse at night, you should analyze what the cause is. This might allow you to achieve better relief of your symptoms.

Helpful hint 2: If your allergies are worse at night, you should consider adjusting the time at which you take your medicine so it coincides with your increased symptoms.

Surprising Death From Bee Pollen

This is a scary story that was reported a few years ago.

Many people take bee pollen capsules in the mistaken belief that bee pollen will cure their allergies. Although certain people claim bee pollen helps, there are no convincing studies that confirm this theory.

My attitude used to be that pollen was cheap. If you felt better using bee pollen, you could use it since you weren't harming yourself, a kind of placebo.

Now, I've changed my mind. Two people had severe allergic reactions and died after using bee pollen.

Bee pollen contains pollen from plants. If you're allergic and ingest substances to which you're allergic, you can suffer massive reactions. In this particular instance, people suffered fatal reactions.

Helpful hint 1: If you're allergic to plant pollens, avoid bee pollen.

Helpful hint 2: There is no convincing research that shows ingesting bee pollen alleviates allergies.

Discovery Of The Worst Location In The United States For Allergy Sufferers

After a short time in practice, I realized that many allergic individuals believe the only reason they're ill with allergy is that they're unlucky enough to be living in the "worst area of the country." This notion isn't correct.

In the United States the incidence of *susceptibility* to allergy is pretty steady at about thirty percent of the population. In fact, this percentage is similar throughout the world. But susceptibility just means you have the *potential* for developing symptoms. Unless you are exposed to *your* allergens, you won't feel a thing. For example, if you are violently allergic to peanuts but never eat them, you won't be ill. If you have asthma when exposed to trees and move to an area which has only grass, you will be asymptomatic. However, if you move to tree country, you will sneeze, cough and wheeze. You'll feel awful. And, if you're like most people, you'll conclude you are living in the worst part of the world for allergy.

And, what do you think a person would say about the worst place for allergy if they are allergic to cats and bring their cats with them when they move? In this situation, *everyplace* is the worst.

Whether you are ill depends on what you're allergic to *and* how much you're exposed to your particular allergens. It's not a specific country, state, or valley.

However, I can disclose, and this may surprise you, that the area of the United States with the highest percentage of allergy is Arizona. Surprised?

Years ago allergy sufferers moved to deserts like Phoenix, Arizona, to escape exposure to pollens. There, they intermarried and had children. Since the ability to make excess IgE antibody is an inherited characteristic, most of their children wound up with the ability to make excessive IgE. In fact, when allergy sufferer married allergy sufferer, they gave their children a double dose of susceptibility.

Then, with irrigation of these desert areas, these allergy sufferers planted trees and grass. And wouldn't you know it, but they planted the very trees and grasses they were trying to avoid in the first place. They also brought their pets. They created dust. Eventually the citizens of Arizona had an environment full of allergenic substances. With so many predisposed people waiting to make IgE antibody and become sick with allergy, you can guess what happened. Arizona wound up with more allergic individuals than other states.

Helpful hint 1: The worst area in the United States is different for different people. This depends on what you're sensitive to *and* what allergens are in your environment.

Helpful hint 2: Because allergy is inherited and because years ago people with allergies moved to Arizona, intermarried, and had children, Arizona now has the highest percentage of allergic individuals in the United States.

Helpful hint 3: If you want to move someplace and a friend tells you it's the worst place for allergies, it may be the worst place for your friend, but this does not mean it will be the worst place for you.

Discovery Of The Worst Year For Allergy Sufferers

When I began practicing allergy, local newspapers and radio stations routinely called my office during the height of the allergy season to ask if this was the worst year I had encountered. I understood their interest because Silicon Valley (Santa Clara County) has a reputation for being the worst area in the country for allergy sufferers. If a reporter could put the worst year together with the worst area, that reporter would have one darn good headline.

I responded to such questions with a complicated answer where I explained about pollen counts, wind factors, availability of medication, and the subjective feeling of patients. I'm sure it sounded like double-talk. As a result, the newspaper journalists never quoted me.

Nevertheless, every year for twenty years a headline would appear stating, "Worst Year Ever According to Dr. So and So." Whenever I saw such a headline, I got this nagging question; How could every year of twenty years be the worst year? One of those twenty years had to be the second worst year. On the other hand, "second worst years" don't sell newspapers.

A few facts which are not of interest to reporters will explain how you judge the severity of a year. One factor is the actual pollen count. The more pollen in the air, the worse the year will be. Second in importance is the strength of the pollen. Depending on the previous year's growing conditions, the various plant pollens will be weaker or stronger. A barrelful of inactive pollen (inactive in allergic terms) cannot compare to a cupful of highly potent pollen.

Third, the wind, rain, barometric pressure and smog level can increase or decrease the severity of allergy symptoms.

Thus, there are *multiple* factors involved. Focusing on only one of them is bound to be misleading. And, trying to assess the severity of a season in the middle of the season *before all the facts are in* is impossible.

The only way to know if a particular year is the worst year in history is to wait until the season ends, count how many people saw allergists compared to previous years, add up the number of prescriptions sold that year, and count the amount of Kleenex people used. Even if allergists seem extraordinarily busy and have patients falling out the windows when the newspaper reporter calls, there could be a sudden change in the weather. The season could end abruptly two days later. However, waiting for the truth is not something newspaper and radio reporters know how to do.

By the way, radio stations and newspapers stopped calling me after a few years. They were not interested in hearing about multiple factors or in waiting until the end of the season. They wanted a yes or no answer right away.

Helpful hint 1: There are many factors that influence how severe a particular allergy season will be.

Helpful hint 2: You cannot tell which is the worst year ever unless you wait until the season ends, count the number of allergy visits during a season, and compare the total to previous years. No one that I know bothers to collect this information.

Helpful hint 3: The true facts of a situation are often not newsworthy.

Treatment For Allergy To X-Ray Contrast Material

When radiologists perform x-ray studies, they often use a substance called radiocontrast material, a chemical that illuminates your interior body organs on x-ray film. Some individuals react to the dye that is used and experience an attack of asthma, hives, or even collapse.

Dr. Roy Patterson's group in Chicago devised a method of circumventing this kind of allergic reaction. Before performing these x-ray procedures, Dr. Patterson gave patients several medications that are known to prevent allergic reactions. The technique has been known for many years, but Dr. Patterson did a service by showing that the procedure is still effective.

Helpful hint 1: If you react to x-ray dye, you can still have X-rays as long as you are pretreated with certain anti-allergy medications.

Latex Glove Skin Reactions

In allergy, repeated exposure leads to sensitivity in susceptible individuals. At the present time, 7 to 10 percent of hospital workers are allergic to latex, which is the material used in most surgical gloves. Even before the AIDS epidemic, hospital personnel wore gloves for sterility. Now these gloves are used routinely outside the hospital, too. Thus many more people are being affected by this condition. And, you can expect many more in the years to come. In fact, if your dentists wear latex gloves while working on your teeth, they may be inadvertently sensitizing you.

Dr. Dennis Ownby of the Henry Ford Hospital even reported that patients who were thought to react to barium used in x-ray studies actually reacted to the latex tubes used to inject barium into the bowel.

At one time it was thought the talcum powder or corn starch used on latex products was the offending agent, but Dr. Alexander Fisher, who is the dean of skin-type allergy, studied this question. He found that the culprits are chemicals in the latex rubber (mercaptobenzothiazole and tetramethylthiuram), and not the rubber itself. This is interesting academically. But, the lesson you need to remember is the same either way: If your skin breaks out when you wear latex gloves, avoid latex.

Helpful hint 1: Sometimes a lot of effort is expended searching for the precise component of an allergenic material when total avoidance is the indicated treatment no matter what component is at fault.

Wife Allergic To Her Husband

Saying you're allergic to your wife or husband is a tired, old joke. However, allergists take everything seriously. And, and lo and behold, Dr. David Bernstein found several women who were truly allergic to their husbands.

In each case, the women broke out in hives, itched all over, and even had shortness of breath and wheezing minutes after having intercourse. Upon investigation, Dr. Bernstein found the women had become allergic to their husband's sperm. After the diagnosis was confirmed by testing, Dr. Bernstein made a special serum, immunized the women with series of allergy injections, and stopped the reactions.

Healthful hint 1: Allergy is an amazing and fascintaing condition that pops up in all kinds of interesting ways.

18

Not New, But
Worth Remembering

There are several topics which aren't new, but you may
not have heard the whole story about them. Since these are
important subjects, I include them here. They unmask
myths that abound in the field of allergy.

The first study describes how a complete allergy history,
all skin tests, and recommendations for treatment can be
completed in little more than an hour. The second study
explains the three types of treatment that are available for
allergies and how each works. Next is an explanation of
why a long series of allergy injections is usually
unnecessary. The fourth study describes the safest way to
use cortisone if you are one of those patients who must use
cortisone. Finally, there is an explanation of the various
types of health care professionals who provide allergy
service. This is humorously titled (at least I think it is
humorous): Will the Real Allergist Please Stand Up?

The One-Visit Allergy Workup

Did you ever wonder why allergists require multiple appointments to diagnose your allergy problem? At the first appointment, they obtain a history. At the next two or three, they perform skin tests. Finally they summarize the results. At some offices, you don't even get to see the allergist until the final visit. A nurse does the work.

When I was in training, we scheduled an hour appointment and completed the workup. This made sense in training, and it still makes sense.

Although it's traditional to have several visits and not dangerous or wrong to do it this way, this tradition costs you extra time and money. There is no scientific reason an allergist cannot take a complete history, do tests by the grouping method (see How to Cut the Cost of An Allergy Workup), and tell you the results on the same day.

Helpful hint 1: There is no medical law that says a complete allergy workup must take multiple visits spread over several weeks.

The Three Treatments For Allergy

One of the most difficult concepts for me to explain is that you must help in selecting your allergy treatment. I wrote about this in *Take Charge of Your Health*, but it's worth repeating some of the facts here.

In many fields of medicine, there is one treatment available. For example, if you have appendicitis, you need an operation. If you have a strep throat, you take an antibiotic. For diabetes, you take insulin.

In allergy, there are nearly always three choices; avoidance, medication, or allergy injections. However, you may be so used to being ordered what to do by your doctors you may be surprised when a health care professional suddenly says you have choices.

Before deciding on a course of *any* treatment, you should understand how that treatment fits *your* situation. For personal, medical, or fanciful reasons, you may prefer one treatment over the other. Your doctors should explain the various options to you.

Let's look at the three allergy treatments. The best treatment is avoidance. This always works, but it is not always practical or possible.

The second method is use of medication. Many drugs are available. And, they work well. But, drugs can produce problems. One problem is they can cause side effects which can be worse than your original symptoms. Common side effects of allergy drugs are nervousness, jitteriness, and drowsiness. Another problem occurs if you take so much medication you build resistance or immunity and the drug stops working. Another problem is that certain drugs don't work. They don't make you better or worse and are a waste of time. The biggest problem with allergy medicine is that no one has invented a medicine that cures allergy. These drugs can relieve your symptoms and make you feel better, but they won't cure you.

The fact that drugs can't cure allergy is not a problem. The drugs for most diseases merely provide symptomatic relief and must be taken continuously. So, allergy drugs are no worse or better in this respect. As you know, doctors don't stop prescribing insulin because it doesn't cure diabetes. They and their patients just realize its limitations.

The third possibility in allergy is the use of immunizing injections. An allergist administers higher and higher doses of a serum which contains allergenic material. This forces your body to make immunity against the substances that trigger your allergy attacks. Using the high dose method, you receive a monthly maintenance dose of serum for about three years. At the end of three years there is generally enough permanent immunity to stop the shots. The schedule may vary depending on the patient, but rarely do you need to be on shots "forever."

In many offices a *low dose* method is used for allergy injections. A patient on the low dose regimen would need more injections, more often, and for more years than I have described. This isn't right or wrong. The low dose just takes longer.

Finally, you have a fourth choice in allergy treatment. This is the drug cortisone. Technically, cortisone could be put in the medication category. I consider it a fourth choice because of the long-term side effects this drug can cause. If you use cortisone, which is a steroid, on a continual basis you risk weight gain, high blood pressure, ulcer, cataracts, softening of bones, stunting growth in children, and psychological changes. To me, steroids should be used *only* when the other measures don't work.

Sometimes it's hard for you to know you are taking steroids. For example, your doctor may prescribe Medrol. You probably wouldn't know that Medrol is a brand of steroid. Or you may be given an "allergy shot" in the nose. Nine times out of ten an allergy shot in the nose is an injection of cortisone. Even a nasal spray may be called by a different name, thus disguising the fact that it is cortisone.

The Allergist's Duty

An allergist's primary job is to help you figure out which of the three choices of treatment would be most suitable *for your particular case.* The answer depends on many factors, but this detective work makes allergy interesting. No two cases are alike. Even if two of you have identical allergies, your treatment might be different because you have different lifestyles.

Helpful hint 1: There are three basic treatments for allergy: avoidance, medication, and allergy injections. Cortisone, the steroid, is a fourth choice because of its serious side effects.

Helpful hint 2: Allergy injections don't have to be taken forever, especially if the high dose method is utilized.

Helpful hint 3: Work cooperatively with your allergists. Be ready to tell them which of the possible treatments fit your situation, which you are willing to follow, and which ones you are reluctant to follow. This will help them decide which path to recommend.

The Best Way To Take Cortisone (Steroids)

Despite the time, money, and effort that has been poured into allergy research throughout the world, there are still hundreds of unanswered questions. The same is true for cardiac disease, cancer, high blood pressure, diabetes, and almost any other illness you can name.

When allergists are stymied for an answer, like most physicians they often turn to steroids. Although steroids can have serious side effects, they also have good effects. In certain situations, the good outweighs the bad.

So, if you reach the point where nothing else is working and your doctor prescribes steroids, there is a hierarchy to follow.

Most desirable method to take cortisone

This first level is tongue in cheek. As I hope you know by now, the best way to take cortisone-type drugs is *not* to take them at all. These compounds can produce long lasting and irreversible side effects. Such problems as cataracts, softening of bones leading to fractures, stunting of growth in children, and thinning of the skin are not uncommon. There are also short-term effects such as weight gain, ulcer, and psychological changes. So, if you can avoid cortisone, do so.

Second best way

If you're still symptomatic after trying the three standard allergy treatments of avoidance, medication, and immunizing injections, your doctor may have no choice but to prescribe cortisone. In that case, begin with a brief burst of cortisone (like one to two weeks of Prednisone, Prednisolone, or Medrol) or a single intramuscular shot (Depo-Medrol). When you use cortisone briefly once a year, this is generally not enough drug to produce the long-term side effects, although the short-term effects could still occur. However, sometimes these brief bursts or shots are repeated frequently. Then, "bursts" turn into the methods described below, even if they weren't intended to.

Third best way

The third best way to avoid long-term side effects (although this may not avoid the short-term effects) is to use cortisone every other day. On the day you don't use cortisone your adrenal gland, the gland that suffers when cortisone is used, has an opportunity to recover. When taking cortisone every other day, it is best to take the whole day's dose in the morning since this further reduces the suppressive effect on the adrenal gland. However, some of you may find taking cortisone once a day is not effective. Then you have no choice but to use it throughout the day to achieve satisfactory relief.

One of the paradoxes of cortisone is that it is manufactured in your adrenal gland. Each night your body measures the amount of cortisone circulating in your bloodstream and makes enough for your next day's needs.

However, your body cannot tell the difference between cortisone that comes from a pill and cortisone it has made itself. So, if cortisone is present in your bloodstream, the adrenal gland figures it doesn't have to make more. When the adrenal gland does not work, it shrinks and atrophies just like your muscle tissue shrinks and becomes flabby when you don't use it.

An atrophied adrenal gland leads to another danger from long-term cortisone use. If you develop a severe infection, need surgery, or suffer stress in which your body needs cortisone-type hormones, your adrenal gland, having been suppressed, is not ready to produce. Atrophied muscles can take months to recover their full strength. Your adrenal gland can take up to a year.

Fourth best way

The fourth best way to take cortisone is to inhale cortisone directly onto your nasal or lung membranes or apply it to your skin. The *theory* is that cortisone will then only affect the local area where it is needed. Distant organs such as bones, muscles, and eyes would be unaffected.

Unfortunately, despite what certain manufacturers claim, cortisone is absorbed from skin surfaces. The more your skin is inflamed and irritated, the more you absorb. When cortisone ointments are applied to your outer skin, from 15 to 30 percent can be absorbed. When it is applied to the thin skin of your eyes, nose, or lungs, an even greater proportion can be absorbed. If your membranes are inflamed, as in the case of allergy, even more is absorbed. Thus, application to your skin does not guarantee protection from *internal* cortisone side effects. Application to the skin is simply equivalent to ingesting a small dose every day.

Dr. John Toogood measured the blood level of cortisone from cortisone inhalers and found enough in the bloodstream to cause weakening of bones (osteoporosis). Dr. H. Bisgaard was able to detect suppression of the adrenal gland when patients used cortisone sprays. Thus both of these doctors have proved that the cortisone in cortisone nasal sprays is absorbed into your body.

Below is a partial list of topical cortisones. A complete list can be found in the *Physician's Desk Reference*, which you can probably find in your local library.

Eye cortisone
  Decadron Ophthalmic
  Inflamase

Nasal cortisone
  Beconase
  Decadron Turbinaire
  Nasacort
  Nasalide
  Vancenase
  Most "allergy shots" which are injected into the nose

Lung cortisone
  Aerobid
  Azmacort
  Beclovent
  Budenoside
  Fluocortin Butyl
  Vanceril

Fifth best way

The fifth possibility is *daily* cortisone. At this point nothing has worked and your doctor's back is against the wall. And, so is yours. Your doctor can start with low doses and then switch you to high doses if necessary. Neither of these are good choices, but when there's no choice, there's no choice. If you must use cortisone daily, you may have to take calcium and in some cases a hormone to prevent weakening of your bones.

After reading the previous five steps, you can well imagine how you can become confused with so many different schedules for taking the same drug. One time you may be told to take cortisone spray, another time a pill every other day, and another time a daily pill.

As you progress from level to level, the specific regimen may seem arbitrary and mysterious. But, there is a logical progression starting with not taking cortisone, going to bursts, progressing to every other day, and finally to daily high doses. I just want you to keep in mind that you and your doctor should do whatever you can to head in the direction of *not* using cortisone.

Helpful hint 1: Cortisone pills, shots, and sprays are not the best thing for your body. Cortisone stops your adrenal gland from functioning and can cause other serious side effects.

Helpful hint 2: When you must use cortisone, there are techniques and regimens to minimize the side effects. We pray that researchers will discover other methods of taking care of allergies so that no one will have to take cortisone in the future.

Helpful hint 3: The reason the dose of cortisone must be tapered when you have been taking cortisone more than a few weeks is to allow your adrenal gland to gradually recoup its strength.

Helpful hint 4: Despite the problems I've described, cortisone is extremely valuable. I wouldn't give it up for anything. It's comforting to know that with a high enough dose, I can relieve almost any allergy problem. In a crisis, this can save a life.

Helpful hint 5: Cortisone is the "no-brain" treatment for allergy. If you don't care what's causing your problem, what side effects you might experience, or what's really underlying your allergy symptoms, use cortisone.

Will The Real Allergist Please Stand Up?

If you need to consult an allergist, you have to choose between certified and uncertified health care professionals. The distinction is based on the amount and thoroughness of training your health care professional obtained when learning to treat allergic diseases.

Since many allergy problems are not complex, you may not require a health care professional who has complete training. In the United States there are only 4,000 professionals anyway. They could not possibly see everyone who has allergy since statistics show that over fifty million people (one-third of the population) have allergy. Thus, chances are high that you will have to obtain your allergy care from someone who has been only partially trained. If your allergy problem is solved, this should not matter.

Like many people you may be embarrassed to ask what kind of training your doctors have and whether they are qualified to handle your case. People who would not hesitate to ask their auto mechanic such questions are too timid to ask when it comes to their own body.

As I mentioned, some allergy problems are obvious and do not require an extensive workup. For example, if you have hives after eating peanuts and a friend tells you to stop eating peanuts, the advice is sound. But, this does not qualify your friend as an allergist.

Beware of Phonies

You must beware of phonies. Because allergy seems like such a simple concept on the surface, there are many health providers who call themselves allergists but who are not trained to do a good job.

Certified Allergists

There are two types of certified allergist, Type I and II. Both must pass an examination in allergy. Then they are called Board Certified in Allergy and Immunology. However, the Type I have had two *additional* years of supervised training in one of fifty special university programs in the United States or Canada while Type II have not. The two years of training come *after* the doctor has already studied three to four years to become a Board Certified Internist, Pediatrician, or Family Practitioner.

You might wonder how a physician could be officially Board Certified but be untrained. In the early nineteen-seventies, there was a separate Board of Allergy for Internal Medicine and Pediatrics. They agreed to merge. At the time, there were many physicians who were practicing allergy but were not considered eligible to take the qualifying examination because they had not gone to one of the special university programs or, in many cases, did not even have the three or four years of training that certified them in Internal Medicine, Pediatrics, or Family Practice.

Despite these physicians' lack of training, a United States court ordered the merged Board of Allergy to allow these physicians to take an examination under a so-called grandfather provision. Many physicians attended cram courses, passed the exam, and thus became Board Certified. If you want to learn whether a person who claims to be a Board Certified Allergist has had the extra two years of training, you may write to the American Board of Allergy and Immunology, University Science Center, 3624 Market St., Philadelphia, PA, 19104.

Remember, untrained physicians can be helpful. Seeing a doctor who has had two extra years of training may not be necessary in your case. Nevertheless you are entitled to a full disclosure of your doctors' background and training so you can make an informed decision. You are entrusting your health to their care.

Uncertified Allergists

There are three types of *uncertified* allergist.

Type III allergists are health care providers such as Family Practitioners, Ear, Nose and Throat Surgeons, Internists, Chiropractors and Acupuncturists. To treat a variety of diseases, these professionals must learn a little about everything, including allergy. Many seminars are held where these health care professionals learn how to assist you.

It's not easy to decide when a problem can be handled by your Family Practitioner, Pediatrician, or Chiropractor, or when you ought to see one of the Type I or II allergists. This is a decision *you* must make. You are the patient who has the problem. You must decide what is in your best interest.

If you are one of the many people who are afraid to hurt your doctors' feelings by asking them for a referral or who assume your doctors would initiate a referral if they felt you needed one, you must overcome those ideas. I have never met doctors who are mad at their patients because patients ask to see a specialist. Many times doctors wait for a patient to request a referral on the assumption that if the symptoms were bothersome the patient would ask. It reminds me of two people who are entering an elevator. Each one waits for the other to go first. Meanwhile the doors close and it's too late for either one to get on.

Type IV allergists call themselves clinical ecologists or environmental allergists. Other ecologists must train them because universities in the United States do not offer this type of instruction. The typical tests (cytotoxic, sublingual, and certain muscle tests) and the typical treatment (injections of chemicals, neutralizing shots, and sublingual drops) that ecologists prescribe have proved to be unreliable in the vast majority of cases. Once in a while a particular patient claims they benefit from ecology treatments. However, when controlled studies are done, the facts hardly ever support the claims.

Even though television and newspapers run articles about this sort of thing, it is extremely rare to find a person who truly has these kinds of allergies. Many individuals react to chemicals in the air. But their reactions are *toxic, irritant* reactions from the excessive levels of fumes, vapors, gases, and particles we must contend with in our industrialized society. This must not be confused with allergy.

Type V allergists are your friends, neighbors, relatives, and pharmacists. Allergy is a common problem. And, everyone seems to have an opinion about it. Sometimes their opinion is correct. Sometimes it is not. You can judge by the results. If a friend's opinion to stop eating peanuts solves your problem, you may not need further advice. If your problem is not solved, you should seek *qualified* help.

Interestingly, the cost of an allergy workup and subsequent treatment is frequently inversely related to the quality and thoroughness of a doctor's training. Type IV ecologists often perform expensive testing using cytotoxic, neutralizing technique, sublingual drops, or total environmental isolation. Their charges can run from $2000 to $10,000. In contrast, charges for a Type I allergist usually run $475 to $600 for a complete workup, including testing and the final summary visit. Type II and III are in-between.

It seems contradictory that doctors who have less training charge more money, but these physicians rely on highly

expensive and inaccurate tests instead of the history,
physical exam, experience, and common sense. Patients
often forget that doing a test is not what is important. It is
the *interpretation* of the test that is important. A blood
pressure of 60/40 might be normal in a small, thin child
who was lying in bed. In an adult, this pressure indicates
cardiovascular shock. A hemoglobin of eighteen might be
normal in an individual who lives on a mountain where
the air is thin. At sea level this indicates a blood disease.

In an era where so many sophisticated tests are available,
you probably want and expect to have the latest ones
performed on you. However, unless you have a scientific
background, you may not be in a position to judge the
usefulness of such tests.

Even doctors are human and can be swayed by advertising
and promotion. Unless your doctors have the time to read
the scientific literature carefully, they can fall into the same
trap as you if you rely on newspaper stories, magazine
articles, and advertising. Food tests are a perfect example.
Skin, blood, sublingual drop, muscle, and neutralizing dose
tests are inaccurate. But they are heavily promoted.
Although these tests are not dangerous, they just don't give
reliable answers. Yet, many physicians may feel pressured
into ordering these tests. And, unaware of the high
frequency of false positive and false negative results, they
may make the mistake of assuming a positive test always
indicates a cause and effect relationship.

I have met Type I allergists who were swayed by the
seductive advertising of companies that promote blood tests
for food allergy. If Type I allergists can be convinced by high
pressure ads, think how easy it is to convince the other
types.

Choosing an allergist is the same as choosing someone to
service your car, television, or taxes. You can go to self-
taught people, those with a moderate degree of training, or
individuals who are fully trained. Whomever you choose,

you may get lucky. But, your chance for a successful outcome is better if you consult someone who has been properly trained.

19

Problems and Deception in Allergy

In allergy, as in other fields of medicine, you need to beware of fraudulent, misguided, or ineffective advice. Whereever you go and whatever you do, you will eventually read and hear about new treatments, drugs, and approaches to common health problems. As you know by now, though, new advice does not automatically mean better advice.

When scientists and researchers propose better ways to heal your body, do not accept their ideas blindly. Ask about the safety and efficacy of each theory, drug, or test. Compare the new proposal to previous and placebo treatments. Then, and only then, consider that treatment for yourself.

Failure to adhere to the above guidelines will result in suboptimal treatment. In the end it is you, the patient, who pays the price.

The first of the following three reports tells you how you can protect yourself when you hear or read of a new treatment, drug, or approach to a health problem. The second report tells you about a recently detected mismanagement problem in allergy which shows how good intentions can go astray. The third describes what many people feel is a typical example of how easy it is to be deceived.

Questions To Ask About A New Treatment Or Theory

Verification of a new theory.
Has the new theory been verified by impartial scientists who confirmed the theory in carefully controlled studies? Or, was the theory verified only by its proponents who would tend to be biased when interpreting the results of the verification tests?

Evaluating claims of opponents of a theory.
If there is a counterclaim that a theory is unproven, does "unproven" mean the theory was proven to be incorrect or does "unproven" mean the theory hasn't been verified? Once a theory has been proven incorrect, that theory should be put to rest. If a theory is untested, you do not want to be the guinea pig to try it.

Evaluating how other patients responded to a treatment.
Did a newspaper article, radio, or advertisement tell you what percentage of people did *not* respond to the new treatment or test? Or, did it only tell you about patients who *did* respond? This kind of reporting can lead you to the false conclusion that the method, drug, or test is guaranteed successful 100% of the time.

Who advocates this theory and what are their credentials?
Did the endorsement come from a television, movie, or sports personality? This might have worked for *them*, but it does not guarantee the method will work for *you*. And unlike them, you are not being paid to use it!

Helpful hint 1: Be careful! For an unwary patient, it's a jungle out there.

Serious Deficiencies That Have Been Noted In The Treatment Of Asthma

Dr. Charles Reed, who teaches at the Mayo Clinic in Minnesota, discovered facts about the treatment of asthma that will astound you.

Doctors have more effective drugs for the treatment of asthma and greater numbers of them than at any time previously. There is deeper understanding of the mechanisms by which asthma produces symptoms. Anyone with common sense would predict that asthmatics must be experiencing fewer symptoms. But, the facts show the opposite!

In the six years from 1977 to 1983, the cost of medicine purchased for asthma shot up two and one half times from 144 million dollars to 362 million dollars (corrected for inflation). Despite the increased use of anti-asthma drugs, the number of patients who had to be admitted to hospitals for asthma doubled from ten to twenty admissions per 10,000 people. How can a country spend twice as much money on advanced drugs and yet have results that are twice as bad?

Scientists analyzed this paradox. They postulated that the increased number of hospital admissions was due to an increased incidence of asthma. But, surveys showed that the number of asthmatics had not changed. Next, they wondered if the problem was peculiar to the United States where it could be blamed on smog, acid rain, or poor diet. But, the identical statistics showed up in other countries, too.

How Can We Be Spending More to Achieve Less?

Dr. Reed didn't know the answer to the above question. Neither do I. But, it's always a challenge to speculate.

One possibility is that patients and doctors rely too much on tests and drugs and therefore ignore the fundamentals of proper allergy treatment. Our society is scientific. And, we often believe more in the power of high technology than in ourselves. For example, you may be one of those who have the impression that medical tests cannot lie since the tests have no feelings or prejudices and can't be influenced by a bad mood, stomach upset, or greed. However, by placing unquestioning faith in tests, you and your doctors may be neglecting the history of your illness. Unless you discuss the when, why, how, and where of your allergy problem, you will likely come to the wrong conclusion.

Talking to Patients Has Gone the Way of the Dinosaur

Both you and your doctors are at fault. When doctors are busy, it is easier for them to give you a prescription for a "new and powerful" drug than to try to convince you to stop smoking or throw your cat out of your house. On the other hand, you may demand "new and powerful" drugs because you don't want to listen to a lecture about stopping smoking or getting rid of your cat.

If asthma statistics were improving, perhaps these considerations would not matter. But the statistics are getting worse. Although I may be considered old-fashioned, I believe that returning to the fundamentals of allergy treatment, which means listening to patients, explaining how to use medication, and discussing proper avoidance, can get all of us back on track to the proper treatment of allergy.

There is a trend toward using video films and slide shows in doctors' offices. I am afraid this is worsening the situation. Busy doctors are thinking, "I know I cannot sit down and talk to each patient as much as I should, so I'll purchase a video. Then, my patients can watch the video in my office. Thus, I'll fulfill my obligations." Although these doctors mean well, they overlook the fact that there is no substitute for a face to face explanation.

When I explain allergy one-to-one, I can tell from my patients' expressions what information they've grasped and what I must repeat in greater detail. Although videos and slides are better than nothing, they are not as effective as a personal instructor.

It's obvious that the new drugs work well. However, unless your doctors explain how to use the drugs properly, as they did with the "old-fashioned" drugs, you will not obtain good results.

When a drug is prescribed for you, you must demand that your doctor explain how to use it. Ask what are its side effects and how long does it take to judge whether it is working. Many new treatments fail not because they are bad but because they are not used properly. For example, in the chapter on nasal sprays, you read that you must use each spray the way it was designed, or there's no point using it at all.

Another explanation for poor results is that many types of health care professional treat allergy (see Will The Real Allergist Please Stand Up?). I've been told it is a matter of opinion what type of doctor is best qualified to help with allergy problems, but it seems to me that an allergist who has spent two extra years studying and specializing in allergy is a better bet.

My third theory for our inability to control asthma more effectively is that the increase in hospital admissions coincided with a swing in the theory of which drug works best for asthma. There are two kinds of asthma drug, theophylline and sympathomimetics. Over the past decade opinion shifted away from the sympathomimetics because they were thought to have excessive side effects. However, these side effects can usually be controlled by adjusting the dose. In the meantime, doctors may have inadvertently created a different problem: fewer side effects but more disease.

Whatever the actual reason for the poor statistics in asthma care, doctors must consider mundane possibilities, like talking more to their patients, and not focus exclusively on expensive research looking for a "new" high-tech drug.

Helpful hint 1: Considering the advances that have been made in the field of allergy, people throughout the world are having more symptoms from asthma than they ought to.

Helpful hint 2: If you have asthma, you are more likely to be treated successfully if you see someone who is well trained to take care of your illness.

Helpful hint 3: A new drug is not necessarily a better drug.

Total Environmental Allergy And Clinical Ecology

Physicians who practice Clinical Ecology or Environmental Medicine have identified a syndrome they call Total Environmental Allergy, or Twentieth Century Syndrome. People who suffer from this disease are said to be allergic to the modern chemicals that surround us at work and home.

Dr. Abba Terr at Stanford University Medical School carefully investigated fifty cases of people who had been told they had this disease. He found nineteen of these people had no disease or just common diseases that are found in the general population such as asthma, hepatitis, conjunctivitis, or hyperventilation.

The remaining thirty-one patients in Dr. Terr's survey had numerous symptoms which involved many different parts of their body. However, their blood, urine, and x-ray tests were normal. There was no evidence of an immune system defect, or even a minor variation in their immune system. In other words, there was no evidence linking their symptoms to allergy or any other immune problem.

Despite the absence of evidence of allergic or immunologic problems, all fifty patients were following treatments recommended by ecologists. Even eight patients who had *no* symptoms at all were obediently following the ecologists' instructions!

These people avoided plastic and synthetic materials at home and work, moved to the country, rigidly observed restrictive rotation diets, and in some cases took allergy injections containing the chemicals they were supposedly allergic to. Dr. Terr found no evidence that any of the recommendations resulted in substantial improvement.

Helpful hint 1: New ideas or theories should never be discouraged or doctors will never learn anything. However, a new theory should be adopted *only* after it has been scrutinized carefully using controlled studies and *only* after the theory has been shown to be correct.

Helpful hint 2: Some patients may benefit from avoidance of synthetic and plastic materials. This makes great headlines and is fun to read and gossip about, but the problem is exaggerated.

Monday Morning Sickness

You've heard of Monday-Morning Blues upon going to work after a relaxing weekend. Now, allergists are confronted with Monday-Morning Flu's.

In certain offices, employees develop flu-like symptoms every Monday morning. At first this was thought to be an allergic reaction caused by something in the workplace environment. Doctors looked high and low but found nothing until they realized they should think of other possibilities besides allergy.

Upon investigating the air-conditioning systems they found bacteria had grown over the weekend and produced toxic chemicals which gushed out when the system went on Monday morning. Cleaning the vents stopped the symptoms.

Helpful hint 1: Although symptoms which occur at the same time and place are usually a certain giveaway to allergy, there are exceptions even to this rule.

20

The Future of Allergy

Many exciting studies hold hope for alleviating allergies. They involve sophisticated research using advanced equipment. Each year another piece of the puzzle falls into place.

No one can predict which, if any, of the current approaches will be the ultimate answer. But the following chapter describes work that is currently in progress.

The first study describes a new substance that has been found to play a role in causing allergic reactions in humans. The hope, of course, is that an antidote could be developed for it.

The second and third studies describe techniques that might stop your body from making excessive IgE antibody.

The fourth study is a science fiction proposal to cure allergy.

Histamine Releasing Factor Has Been Found To Be Responsible For Allergies

One of the most intensely studied subjects in allergy is how chemical mediators provoke the actual symptoms you experience.

For years doctors have known that histamine is one of the most important chemical mediators that contribute to allergic reactions. The antidote, antihistamine, ameliorates the symptoms by acting *after* histamine is already released into your tissues from cells called Mast cells. Wouldn't it be better if doctors could prevent histamine from being released in the first place?

Now, researchers have a better chance to accomplish this feat. They have discovered a substance called Histamine Releasing Factor. As the name implies, Histamine Releasing Factor is responsible for releasing histamine into your tissues. If pharmacolgists can find a drug to block the effect of Histamine Releasing Factor, this could lead to a major advance in allergy treatment.

Unfortunately it can take a long time for pharmaceutical manufacturers to develop effective drugs. Even when they do, the drug must be tested for dangerous side effects. But it's good to know that scientists have not given up the search for basic answers to allergy problems.

Exciting And Revolutionary Treatment For Allergies

At a patient's first office visit, I explain the three methods of treating allergy: avoidance, medication, and allergy injections. I also mention the last hope, and fourth choice, cortisone. Now Dr. Kimige Ishizaka, who was the first scientist to isolate IgE antibody in quantity and show that

IgE was the root cause of allergy, has discovered a chemical in rats which prevents the rats from making IgE antibody. He calls it GIF which stands for glycosylation inhibiting factor.

GIF is one of a family of chemicals called Interferon. It activates certain immune cells which can then suppress the production of IgE antibody.

It is years and years too early to become optimistic about GIF. Many experiments have to be performed to confirm these initial findings. Also, we must learn whether Dr. Ishizaka's discoveries apply to humans as well as rats. And lastly, doctors must determine whether GIF is safe to use in humans. Nevertheless, someone has finally opened a crack in the door to getting directly at the manufacture of too much IgE, which is the fundamental malfunction that leads to allergy.

Helpful hint 1: Dr. Kimige Ishizaka has found a substance that may be able to turn off the manufacture of excessive IgE antibody and thus cure allergy.

Another New Treatment For Allergy

Like Dr. Ishizaka, Dr. Alec Sehon of Canada has been able to turn off IgE production in animals. He attached various allergenic proteins to a chemical called polyethylene glycol (PEG). When he injected his creation into laboratory animals, they stopped making IgE antibody for that particular allergen.

If this is going to be useful, doctors have to figure out how to attach allergens to polyethylene glycol in a safe way so that this new chemical does not create a worse disease in humans than it was meant to prevent.

A Science-Fiction Proposal For An Allergy Cure

This is a science-fiction proposal that could cure allergy with just a few injections.

As you know by now, allergy is caused when excess IgE antibody is attached to Mast cells. If doctors could remove the IgE from cells, they could prevent allergic symptoms from occurring. Unfortunately, removing antibodies while they are in your body is technically difficult. However, *replacing* them with another chemical is feasible.

The best substitute for IgE would be an *inactive* IgE molecule. The inactive, or false, IgE could attach to the cells, blockade the existing sites, and, being inactive, would be incapable of causing a reaction itself. Furthermore, inactive IgE is merely a modification of natural IgE and would not be a foreign chemical that might cause all sorts of undesirable side effects.

The ideal chemical for this job is the end portion of the IgE molecule itself. This portion, which is called the "Fc fragment" of IgE is the segment of the molecule that specifically binds to IgE sites and no other sites. Therefore, the Fc fragment fulfills all the criteria for our science fiction proposal.

• The Fc fragment is a specific component of a natural substance that is already found in the body. So, it is not a foreign drug.

• The Fc fragment has a strong attraction for IgE sites (scientists call this strong attraction a "high affinity"), and it is known to stick to the IgE site for long periods of time so it would not have to be replaced every few hours or even every few days.

• Finally, and most important, the Fc fragment is inactive. Thus, it could not trigger allergic reactions on its own.

Below is a diagram showing you how this might work.

The IgE molecule is made up of two sections. The Fc fragment is the tail and the Fab fragment is the head. If the whole IgE molecule looked like this,

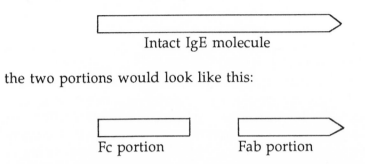

Intact IgE molecule

the two portions would look like this:

Fc portion   Fab portion

If your doctors flooded your body with blunted, inactive Fc fragments, these would bind to your Mast cells. Without a pointed Fab end, though, these molecules cannot grab onto grasses, weeds, or dust allergens. Since the allergens cannot attach to Mast cells via the IgE antibody, they would float by and be unable to trigger the release of chemical mediators like histamine. This would prevent allergic reactions.

To my knowledge, no one has done this successfully. But with the current plethora of genetic research and the amazing creation of chemicals through gene splicing, this should be possible.

A Final Word

I hope you enjoyed reading *What's New in Allergy,* and I hope the information helps you overcome your allergy problems. However, no book can anticipate all questions. So, consult your doctors and make them part of your anti-allergy team.

Appendix A

Partial List of
Drugs Used in Allergy

This is a partial list of the drugs used for the treatment of allergic disorders. Each drug is listed according to whether it is old, new, or super-new. If you would like a complete list of drugs, you can find it in the suggested reading in Appendix B.

Decongestants

Old

phenylephrine
phenylpropanolamine
phenyltolaxime
pseudoephedrine

Antihistamine (many contain decongestants)

Old
  Atarax
  Benadryl
  Chlortrimeton
  Naldecon
  PBZ
  90 others

New
  Astemizole
  Hismanal
  Seldane
  Tavist
  Terfenadine
  Trinalin

Super-New
  Cetirizine
  Ebastine
  Ketotifen
  Levocbastine
  Loratidine
  Mequitazine
  Noberastine
  Oxatomide
  Pemirolast
  Seldane-D

Sympathomimetic Bronchodilators

Old
: adrenalin
ephedrine
Isoproterenol
Isuprel
Susphrine

New
: Albuterol
Brethaire
Bricanyl
Brethine
Maxair
Metaprel
Proventil
Salbutamol
Terbutaline
Ventolin

Super-New
: Berotec
Bitolterol
Fenoterol
Formoterol
Lanetolol
Procaterol
Rotocaps
Salmeterol
Tornolate
Turbohaler

Theophylline Bronchodilators

Old   Choledyl
                 Marax*
                 Quibron
                 Slobid
                 Slophyllin
                 Tedral*
                 Theo Dur
                 Uniphyl

*also contains a sympathomimetic

Steroids

Old
Aristocort
Decadron
Kenalog
Medrol
Prednisolone
Prednisone

New
Azmacort
Beclomethasone
Beclovent
Beconase
Flunisolide
Nasalide
Triamcinolone acetonide
Vancenase
Vanceril

Super-New
Budenoside
Fluocortinbutyl
Fluticosone propionate
Nasacort

Anti-allergic

Old	Disodium Cromoglycate
	Intal
New	Gastrocrom,
	Nasalcrom
	Opticrom
Super-New	Lodoxamide Tromethamine
	Nedocromil
	Rhinocrom
	Tiprinast
	RO22-3747*
	Tranilast
	Amlexanox

*also known as trans-3-[6-(methylthio)-4-oxo-4H-quinazolin-3-yl]-2-propenoic acid

Atropine-like

Old	Atrovent
	Ipratropium Bromide
	SCH-1000

Appendix B
Other Books About Allergy

There are many books on the subject of allergy. You should talk to your doctors and visit your local library. The ones I mentioned in this book are described below.

Hidden Food Allergies; How To Find And Overcome Them Successfully by Stephen Astor, M.D.

Hidden Food Allergies describes a seven step process that will enable you to determine whether you have food allergy. If you find that you suffer from food reactions, you will then learn how to pinpoint the offending food and how to overcome the problem. This book contains hints about coping with food allergy, a section with allergy-free recipes, and a section which lists groups of allergically-related foods.

Published by Avery Press $7.95;

Take Charge of Your Health by Stephen Astor, M.D. ($12.95)

Does your doctor listen to you? Do you understand the treatments you take? Are you in control of your own health? This is not some New Age guilt trip that tells you sickness is in your head and that if you don't get better it's your own fault. Rather, it is a practical guide for patients (and health care professionals) who don't approve of the offhand manner in which medical advice is often given. This insider's view of health care in America offers all the tools readers need to become the decision maker where their health is concerned.

Published by Two A's Publishers; (available from Two A's Publishers, 285 South Drive, Mountain View, CA 94040-4318 for $14.95 including postage and handling).

Take Charge of Your Allergy by Stephen Astor, M.D. (Available Summer 1992)

Take Charge of Your Allergy describes the practical steps to overcome allergy. This book explains what drugs are used for allergy treatment, teaches you how to choose the medication that is best for you, describes the modern efficient way to avoid various allergens, and explains when to consider allergy injections.

The Best Guide to Allergy by A. Giannini, M.D., N.Schultz, M.D., T. Chang, M.D.

This book has an easy to follow question and answer format. Published by Consumer Reports books.

INDEX

Additives, food, 19
Adrenaline, 56, 153,166
Air cleaners, 143
  electrostatic, 143
  HEPA, 143
Albuterol, 56, 65, 89
Allergist,
  certified, 171
  uncertified, 172
Allpyral, 67
Antihistamine, 57
  categories, 79
  long acting, 82
  for asthma, 76
Arthritis, 30
Aspartame, 135
Aspirin, 21
Astemizole, 82
Asthma, 20, 76, 103
  delayed, 103
  deficiencies in treatment,
    179
  exercise, 113
  pregnancy,119
Adrenal gland, 166
Atropine, nasal spray, 97

Bee pollen, capsules, 153
Bee sting, 130
Beta blocker, 92
Binders, 13
Bisulfite, 20, 106
Blood tests, 48
  for foods, 48
Breast feeding, allergy
  prevention, 9

Cat allergy, 34
Certified allergist, 171
Clinical Ecology, 173, 182
Coating, 13
Coloring agents, 13
Colors, 13
Cortisone, nose spray,
  96
Cortisone, 58
  how to take, 165
Cromolyn, 27
  nasal spray, 97
Cytotoxic Test, 48, 173

Decongestant spray, 94
Delayed asthma, 103
Disintegrant, 13
Dog allergy, 34
Drug reaction, types, 83
Drugs, how to take, 88
Dust mites, 68, 141
Dust, house, 141

Electrostatic, air cleaner, 143
ELISA, 50
Eosinophils, 139
Epinephrine, 56
Exercise wheezing, 112
Exercise, 112, 114, 134

False negative, 174
False positive, 174
Feingold, Dr. Ben, 21
FICA test, 49

Fillers, 13
Flavors, 13
Food, allergy, 25, 45
  delayed, 45
  immediate, 45

Gastrocrom, 29
Glidant, 13

Hamsters, 34
Hayfever, 149
HEPA, 143
Histamine Releasing Factor,
  186,
Histamine release test, 48
Histamine, 15
Hives, 133, 138
  chronic, 135
Hyperactivity, 21

Idiosyncratic reaction, 83
IgE, 14
Immunizing drops, 70
Immunizing injection, 57,163
Immunizing injections, for
  animals, 36
Inhalers, 109, 110
Insulation, 144
Interleukin, 15
Intolerance, 83
Ion generator, 111

Kapok, 141
Ketotifen, 89
Killer bees, 131

Lactose intolerance, 28
Late onset reaction, 103
Latex allergy, 159
Local Nasal Immunotherapy
  (LNIT), 98
Lubricant, 13

MAST test, 50
Medicators, chemical, 11, 14
Metered dose inhaler, 108
Methacholine test, 105
Migraine, 31
Milk allergy, 30
Minor Determinant Mixture,
  126, 12
Molds, 40, 70
Motrin, 20

Naprosyn, 20
Nasal spray, 94

Occupational allergy, 1365
Oral immunizing, 70
Overdose, 83

Paradoxical asthma, 107, 116
Penicillin, 123
  tests for, 125
Perforation, nasal, 99
Polyethylen glycol, 12, 187
Polymerized serum, 60
Pregnancy, 119
Priming, 150
Prostaglandin, 15
Provocation test, 47

Radiocontrast material, 158
Ragweed, 69
RAST, 48
Rhinitis, 138

Salt water, 94
Seldane, 80
Serum, allergy, 66
Side effect, 83
Sinus disease, 105, 148
Smoking, 115
Spacer, 109, 110
SRS-A, 15
STALLERZYM, 50
Steroids, 165
Sublingual test, 47
Sugar, allergy, 26
Sulfite, 21
Sus-Phrine, 56
Sweeteners, 13
Systemic reaction, 130

Tagamet, 77
Terbutaline, 56
Testing, allergy, 44
  need to repeat, 71
Theophylline, 86, 88
  blood test for, 87
Treatments for allergy, 162
Twins, 8

Uncertified allergist, 172

Venom, 120
Vitamin C, 84

Vitamin, 12

Yellow food dye, 20

Coming in Fall 1992

Take Charge of Your Allergy and Asthma

Ordering Information

To order, send the following information to:

Two A's Industries, Inc.
285 South Drive   Suite 1
Mountain View, CA   94040-4318

Name:_____
Address:_____
_____
Phone #:_____

Check or money order made payable to: Two A's Industries, Inc. Prices include shipping.

Indicate which book you want;

	California addresses	Non-California addresses
What's New in Allergy	14.50	13.50
Take Charge of Your Health	15.50	14.50

Surface Shipping may take three to four weeks. If you prefer air mail, add $3.00 per book.

Payment:
Payment must be made by check or money order. <u>Do not send cash</u>.